MRSA, MRSA Me!

A First Person Story

of Gross Negligence Medical Malpractice,

the Lawsuit which Followed,

Thoughts on Fighting Back and Reform

David L. Folck

TRUE STORY PUBLISHERS

MRSA, MRSA Me!
A First Person Story of Gross Negligence Medical Malpractice,
the Lawsuit Which Followed, Thoughts
on Fighting Back and Reform
by David L. Folck

Copyright 2013 by David L. Folck

Printed in the United States of America.

First Printing 2013

ISBN: 978-1484870297

True Story Publishers
549 Appleton Road
Simi Valley, CA 93065
Website: http://mrsamrsame.com

Should you have your head examined before filing a medical malpractice lawsuit?

Table of Contents

Author's Note

In June 2011, while waiting for a right shoulder arthroscopy at (pseudonym) Valleydale Hospital Medical Center (VHMC) in (pseudonym) Valleydale, California, City of Los Angeles (true), Los Angeles County (true), I was reminded of my awful med mal experience. The trigger was that I had been singled out on that morning for having a history of a serious bacterial infection at VHMC beginning in March 2004. It was ironic that they were singling me out when seven-plus years earlier this very same medical center had initially bungled the notification to me of my infection, and bungled it royally.

What they were attempting to do with me was important since the bacteria in question could be spread by human contact to another human or by human contact to an inanimate object and then contact with the infected object to another human being. While aware of this, I was reminded at the same time of all that I had been through because of the negligence of other individuals.

*****

According to John A. Nyman and a 2011 study, by eliminating the bacteria after it is detected in U.S. patients entering a hospital, expected cost savings would be between $3.2 and $4.2 billion annually.[i]

According to Dr. Ramanan Laxminarayan and Dr. Anup Malani, hospital-acquired sepsis and pneumonia, which are often linked to MRSA as well as other hospital-acquired infections, cost the United States $8 billion to treat in 2006.[ii]

*****

Most of the time, I am not prone to displays of anger. They are very few and far between in my life. However, the subject of the bacterial infection at that time was too much for me to take passively. Also, I am not one to just sit quietly when I think someone is picking on me, and I felt that I was being picked on that morning.

When it was thrown in my face, I lashed out at the person who brought it up — swearing and screaming at her in an awful tone of voice ready to fight her to the death. She put her hand on me to try to calm me down and I screamed at her not to touch me as I knocked her hand away.

It upset me very much to be reminded of that earlier life-threatening situation. That was the impetus to pull out some notes and files I had compiled in 2007 and to attempt to complete this project — that is, to write a book about my med mal experience. Yes, I had failed on my first attempt to write it back in 2007 as I became totally overwhelmed recalling everything. But this time, over two years, I was able to complete the book you are now reading.

A One-Sided, Outdated System

After surviving the medical malpractice, I endured the California medical malpractice legal system. *That* was a very dissatisfying experience, which left me extremely depressed.

Because of that, the one-sided, outdated system of legal remedies in California for medical malpractice cases was placed under my microscope. The current California med mal law was enacted by elected officials more than thirty-seven years ago during a so-called "medical malpractice insurance crisis." It was never a ballot initiative. It was enacted without much concern for injured patients and a lot of concern for doctors potentially going out of business due to rapidly rising medical malpractice insurance premiums, which might have created a shortage of available medical care.

In this country, medical malpractice insurers are hiding a secret from the public at large. Within these pages, you will read evidence which will support that prior sentence. By the end of the book, you will come to clearly understand what is meant by the word "secret."

The people responsible for the malpractice control the information about malpractice injuries and, essentially, no government agency checks on this information which appears in a patient's records, except if someone questions it. If there are checks and balances, they are not universal. If reporting occurs at all, only the most serious medical malpractice cases are reported. And punishment for the wrongdoers may never come or may seem unsatisfactory.

Vital Information

I hope that you will read the entire book. If you don't, you will miss some vital information — especially about medical malpractice reform — that is both timely and necessary. If you don't read these pages, you simply *will not* understand why I saw some of the things the way I did and why I wrote what I did.

No one in his or her right mind would want to write about the personal misfortune and anguish of a medical negligence injury. **But I did**.

If my efforts help to change the present system for the better and/or keep one person from getting clobbered like I did, I will feel wildly successful. I didn't write this to cry in my beer, nor to be a hero. I wrote it to open people's eyes.

*****

Several of the names used in the story are pseudonyms and were used due to privacy issues or potential legal issues that might arise against me.

Introduction

There was no way I thought that certain events in my life, which began in late December 2003, would ever be the subject of a book. However, what occurred, beginning back then, became too much for me to keep inside.

What I wrote in the pages that follow is not a blood and guts tale of "they done him wrong" but rather an introspective look at a personal nightmare. It is every man's worst fear coming true.

The story that follows is a first-person account of an awful experience in my life, what caused it to happen, and the heavy price I paid. I already had two serious medical conditions on my plate when the third medical crisis hit.

Other books have been written about medical malpractice over the years. None that I am aware of follow a first-person account of a medical malpractice experience. THIS ONE DOES.

In writing the book, which is intended to be a case study, I sought to:

1. Share an actual medical malpractice case from a first-person point of view;

2. Detail what might happen in a medical malpractice case legally and what did happen in my case;

3. Point out flaws in the laws governing medical malpractice cases;

4. Suggest changes to medical malpractice laws that are sorely needed;

5. Find some peace of mind for myself.

In no way do I want you to perceive me as a martyr as you read this. It happened and I lived through it.

Other Points of View Needed

Why should you be interested in a book about medical malpractice?

In his State of the Union address in 2011, President Barack Obama singled out medical malpractice reform. The President indicated that he would consider other ideas to bring down healthcare costs, and he identified medical malpractice reform as one area to look at, alluding to frivolous lawsuits.[iii]

Referring to President Obama's remarks, the Congressional Budget Office (CBO) estimated that savings to Medicare and Medicaid by capping non-economic damage awards (known as *pain and suffering*) for injured patients would be about $50 billion over nine to ten years.[iv]

The CBO report says nothing about the economic realities to injured parties from capping non-economic damages. It is strictly a single-number argument for macro-management. The fallout of such a strategy is a major topic in this book.

One of the major concerns in the United States today for its residents and leaders is HEALTHCARE. That makes this book part of a major story.

Steven Brill, writing in the March 14, 2013 issue of *Time* magazine, said that the culprits in high medical costs are federal laws, greedy hospitals and medical facilities, greedy medical equipment manufacturers and suppliers, greedy medical service providers, and the way hospitals and healthcare facilities price products and services.[v]

Medical malpractice potential cost savings to the federal government are miniscule compared to the hundreds of billions in potential savings from reigning in federal healthcare costs and healthcare costs in general, according to Brill's numbers. In other words, the feds are barking up the wrong tree.

The Shocking Truth

Medical injuries are very personal when they are preventable. Medical malpractice injuries are extremely difficult to deal with physically and emotionally.

That was what galled me the most about what happened to me, that my injury was *preventable*. That made it a serious violation of a very significant personal trust, the trust between a seemingly competent physician and a patient. In my case, more than one physician and a medical center were involved.

This is not a story about the worst case of medical malpractice negligence that ever occurred. It is offered as a backdrop to a larger story, which is the *shocking truth* about medical malpractice in this country and *the lies* that are perpetuated about it. The lies perpetuate a myth that does not allow all those injured by medical malpractice to obtain justice under current laws.

A Call for Meaningful Reform

As I delved into the current state of medical malpractice laws in California and the United States, my curiosity lead me on a search for meaningful medical malpractice reform. Time and space did not permit a lengthy discussion on that topic, so only a brief, informative, eye-opening summary is included.

As you will come to learn, there is nothing "frivolous" about filing a valid medical malpractice lawsuit. The burden of proof is very high for a med mal plaintiff in California and in many other states.

Who Should Read This Book

As I wrote these pages, I saw that the information would provide critical insights to many different types of readers.

For any federally elected official contemplating medical malpractice reform: You need to read this book before you do something shallow and narrow-minded regarding med mal reform. You need to grasp *what is really going on with med mal* before you act.

If you are contemplating filing a medical malpractice lawsuit in California, or if you have already filed one, you should read this book. Even if you are contemplating filing a med mal lawsuit outside of California, you should read this.

Should you be a licensed medical professional, a medical school student, a medical resident or intern, a hospital administrator, hospital staff member or infectious disease control specialist, you need to read this book.

If you are an attorney, law school student, paralegal, state legislator, governor, consumer rights advocate or reporter who covers medical/legal issues, you need to read this book.

Lastly, if you are interested in the quality of healthcare, work for a medical insurance carrier, work for a medical malpractice insurance company, or you are interested in medical malpractice reform, you need to read this book.

Prologue

What people, life events, personal experiences, teachings and personality traits helped me to endure a near-death experience and the aftermath?

I had a schema to follow as this story began and then fully developed because I was fortunate to have had the mother that I did.

During the writing process, I was also incredibly fortunate to have the imagination that I possess. I also summoned a multi-faceted sense of humor that helped me a great deal.

According to my Meyers-Briggs Test results, I am the classic **Intuitive-Thinker** or INTJ. That means that my strongest personality traits are my intuition and my ability to think. Those come to the forefront in times of need.

My IQ is between 135 and 140. Because of that, I am able to understand *how **many** things work* — including medical procedures — and how medical conditions evolve.

Lastly, I don't give up easily.

My Mom, Marilyn

My mother, Ruth Marilyn (Melcher) Folck, was my sole parent beginning in August 1952. I was just three and a half years old when my father, Jean D. Folck, who was a heavy equipment operator, died at work.

Prior to Dad's death, some people in the maintenance department at the Sunflower Ordnance Company in Ottawa, Kansas didn't think it was important enough to maintain the hydraulic system on the tracked shovel my father was operating. As he drove it above a ravine along a narrow lane on his last day alive, the road started to give way. Dad tried to stop but the brakes failed, and he and the machine were smashed into pieces after falling into the ravine.

Years later, when Mom finally told me this, I realized that this incident was the first one that adversely affected my life due to negligence. I asked her, "Why didn't you sue the bastards?!"

My mother said that she never pursued a lawsuit because the thought of it was too gut-wrenching for her. She turned the other cheek over his death. Personally, had it happened to one of my loved ones, I would have come out with six guns blazing at the offenders.

In trying to explain the situation to me, Mom told me that God must have wanted my dad very badly. My response to that was "I needed him more than God did."

The daughter of a civil engineer and a high school English teacher, Marilyn was an RN. She had a BS in Nursing from the University of Iowa (graduating in 1943) and an MSN from UCLA (graduating in 1957). She revered higher education.

Because of that, I was very aware of things medical — at least more so than most other people my age as I grew up.

The Kidney Infection

What happened to me in March and April of 2004 was not my first medical crisis. That happened when I was ten years old in 1959.

Unbeknownst to me, I had developed a kidney infection as a side effect of the Asian flu that was making the rounds that year. It went undetected and untreated because of an incompetent doctor, the first one that I ever encountered.

The infection had some nasty side effects. Occasionally, I had tarry stools, a little bit of blood after urinating, and a frequency to urinate that drove me crazy **for years**.

After having me as a patient for approximately six months, the "doctor" concluded that my symptoms were all in my head. This was in spite of the objective evidence to the contrary. He was from Harvard Medical School.

Mom took me to the Marion Davies Children's Clinic at UCLA six months after I first showed symptoms of this medical problem, and they diagnosed the kidney infection with a lighted probe inserted in my penis under anesthetic. After that, I had to be on a sulfa-based antibiotic for six months.

The medication made me feel tired, and I could only attend school for half-days. I also felt like I had to pee frequently until I was fourteen years old, as a psychological side effect of the infection. I had been conditioned to pee frequently and it took all that time for the feelings to subside.

My mother never got me any psychotherapy to get past those awful feelings, even though her specialty was psychiatric nursing. *Go figure.* In 1959, psychotherapy was not as common as it is today.

At one point before the infection was discovered, an x-ray technician at UCLA got my x-rays mixed up with those belonging to another pediatric patient. As a result, my mother was told that I had an inoperable brain tumor. Emotionally, she lost it. Two days later, she was informed of the mix-up. However, during those two days, my mother, despite medical evidence that I had a urinary tract problem, lost her precious objectivity. How does one get tarry stools and blood in their urine and a frequency to pee from a brain tumor?

I heard about this from Mom for the first time when I was fifty years old.

I became pretty much of a solitary person in so many ways from that kidney infection and the aftermath. I didn't tell a soul about it as it was *so* embarrassing. I learned to keep things inside and not to talk about them. I learned not to talk about my feelings. I spent much of my adult life from age forty on trying to undo that.

As I recovered from the kidney infection, my mother told me that sometimes men just had to get over things. In other words, you just had to suck it up in this life and keep going. She said that during their lives, men experience difficult events and they just have to put their thoughts aside. Remember, she was trained to be a public health nurse and later a psychiatric nurse. Yet when it came to her two sons, they would just have to suck it up in this life.

"No!" to Football

My mother also acted in protective ways at times. However, it was to protect *her* more than my brother or me. She could not stand the idea of either son getting seriously injured in some way on her watch. Mom openly resisted us playing sports, especially football. We were both very big in our high school years.

My mom made me conscious of my size as I grew up. She wanted a gentle big man and not some testosterone-filled hot head in the family. I was fairly shy as a child partly because of this.

I was so large at birth compared to others and I stayed that way all my life. Yet she thwarted my efforts to play high school football. Defiantly, on at least three occasions, she said, "I won't allow it!"

Even when I said I would buy my football shoes and pay for the insurance, the answer was "No!"

Mom's Strong Personality

At one time, Marilyn taught undergraduate nursing students at UCLA. She later retired as the Chief Nurse (like the Director of Nursing) for the County Mental Health Services in San Diego.

That's right; **I was raised by a real-life Nurse Ratched**. Louise Fletcher's movie character couldn't hold a candle to my mom. Talk about disciplined and at times overbearing — that was Marilyn. By the time my brother and I were in our late teens, we had had enough of Marilyn's ways.

My mom spoke many times about "The Big Lie." She pointed out examples all the time. Politicians told "The Big Lie," so did corporations, lawyers and many others with something to hide or gain something by lying. She said, "Watch out for them. They'll get you." I learned that first hand, especially during my military service. I saw it in the business world as well.

Marilyn was very good at discerning the central issue regarding just about any topic. She called it "The Elephant." She said, "If you miss it or fail to grasp it, whatever decisions you make after that are likely to be bad. Don't miss **the elephant**." We would discuss examples of this at length as I grew up.

An Accidental Injury

In November 1984, I tore the meniscus in my left knee while managing a store for Chief Auto Parts. Because of that injury and a subsequent injury to the same knee, I went into a deep depression and did not work for several years. It was my first experience with an accidental injury leading to a severe depression, but it would not be my last.

I filed a worker's comp lawsuit and prevailed. It was the first lawsuit I ever filed.

The Ruptured Appendix

When my son Darrell was eleven, I drove him to play in an all-star baseball game in Santa Susana Knolls in Simi Valley. We traveled from Mission Hills in the San Fernando Valley via the 118 Freeway, about fifteen miles. I didn't know it at the time, but my appendix ruptured as I drove through the Santa Susana Pass. I almost passed out from the pain but got Darrell to his baseball game. Then I went to Valley Presbyterian Hospital in Van Nuys, where I stayed for a week recovering from an appendectomy. This was in June 1986 and at that time the bill for the antibiotics alone was $18,000 since I was septic. That was my first near death experience in a medical sense. From that experience I knew that no matter what, I had to keep going.

Two days before my appendix ruptured, I went to the ER at Valley Presbyterian Hospital for severe abdominal pain. The female ER doctor never once touched my lower right abdomen on that visit but prescribed antacid for me to treat my pain. Talk about medical malpractice. I wonder if she is the director of a hospital Emergency Room these days.

The "Baby Central" Dream

At times in the last twenty-five years, I've had a recurring dream. It has to do with the events immediately preceding my birth. The dream goes something like this:

An imaginary cast of characters at "Baby Central" selects me to come into the world programmed to deal with major adversity all through my life. The "Boss" at Baby Central, a cigar-chomping, suspender-wearing, bespectacled, paunchy middle-aged man named Max, says I am a tough kid and that I will be able to "take it."

One of Max's assistants says that with all the strife on the horizon for me, all of it will do me in at a young age. Max disagrees and feels that weathering it will make me a strong, resourceful, self-reliant person.

"Baby Central" is a mythical place in the clouds that I have fantasized about to explain the myriad of inexplicable perilous situations permeating my life at different times. Imagining it has brought me peace of mind. It has helped me to move on through difficult times.

Support for the Journey

All of the things mentioned above aided me greatly. But my Mom deserves most of the kudos. She taught me that my body, my mind, my education, my life experiences, and my life are very precious.

So there you have it. These were the major life experiences, teachings and personality traits that I drew upon during the course of this story. As it turned out, I needed all of them.

Part I: My Medical Nightmare

Chapter 1—April 12, 2004

No other day I have experienced has matched that of April 12, 2004. It was a day that would change my life forever and have lasting consequences.

How did it feel to be dying from the effects of a virulent, deadly bacterial infection? After dredging up nightmarish memories regarding how I felt on that fateful day, I've come to the conclusion that I felt awful in every way.

The only thing that was good about that day was that I lived through it.

Since March 27, 2004 until the day in question, my life had been hell. I had been told by two medical doctors and a resident physician during that time that I was receiving the proper medication for what ailed me.

Hell, one of the doctors was adamant about what ailed me — "bronchitis." Not knowing anything to the contrary, I believed this.

Bronchitis usually is not fatal. Though I felt terrible, I had no reason to be morbidly concerned about my condition. After all, what reasons did I have to doubt two experienced physicians and a resident who concurred with each other about the treatment of my maladies? At least that is what I was told.

Meanwhile, a golden-hued bacterium, which formed in grape-like clusters as seen under a microscope, was permeating evil on my body. I would later learn that this was a fairly common bacterium most of the time. However the strain I had was rare.

Most often, when the bacterium in question was detected, it hardly caused a stir among medical professionals. A regimen of an appropriate antibiotic usually eliminated it from one's body with no permanent damage done. Treating it was like putting an airplane on auto-pilot.

Unfortunately, my case was not a regular case. No, this was the type of case that professors bring up in medical school lectures to point out that this bacterium could have potentially ruinous consequences — if left unchecked or if **the wrong medication** was used to treat it.

My saving grace would be a radical intervention of the most serious kind. It would take sharp, experienced medical minds to pull me out of my decline, unlike the two doctors who had been treating my condition.

*****

A little background. The bacterium in question — *Staphylococcus aureus* — was first observed by Dr. Alexander Osmong in 1880 in Scotland according to Wikipedia. He looked at pus from post-surgical abscesses and saw the bacteria with a microscope.

Over the years, this bacteria has successfully dodged, bobbed and weaved from successive new generations of antibiotics as it wreaked havoc on the human race. Some strains of the bacteria developed a resistance to penicillin or penicillin-based drugs.

*****

Exponentially worsening over time, the bacteria within my body was pushing the life out of me. In the condition I was in, it had several possible ways to do me in: a stroke; a heart attack; or a pulmonary embolism.

My breathing was quite labored that momentous day, April 12th. With every passing day since March 27th, it had become harder to breathe. I had forgotten what "normal" breathing felt like.

Along with the symptoms of my "bronchitis," my sleep was torched. I was a man who needed decent sleep for a variety of reasons which you will discover later on.

My brain was in a fog-like state caused by severe clinical depression. Actually, I had been diagnosed with it, long before, in 1992, and had displayed symptoms of it since 1969. It had reared its head too often in my adult life.

Also, icy, full-body, shivering chills made me shake all over, due to the bacteria. In contrast, a high fever caused me to sweat bullets of perspiration.

The breaks between the cycles of chills and fever were getting shorter over time. My condition showed itself and then hid itself, which is typical. But only a highly skilled physician could surmise that and only with some confirmation.

With all that was going on with my health, I had little time for normal thoughts or regular activities of daily living. I was just trying to make it through the day about an hour at a time. Then I would focus on getting through the next hour.

The coughing was the worst. As big as I am, I felt that I could launch a lung from my body through my mouth with the unrestrained force I had behind the coughs.

"What in the hell is going on?" I wondered.

You see, the information I had on my medical condition was incomplete. I had only gotten bits and pieces.

It wasn't that I hadn't tried very hard to learn what ailed me. Repeated visits to two doctors, lab test results, and knowledge that I had a blood infection still left me wondering what I was dealing with.

Could it be that some people that I trusted were ignoring the obvious?

*****

On April 10th, I had been switched off one ineffective antibiotic and **prescribed one that was supposed to work better**. I was told to go to a hospital ER by an internist who was treating me. Instead, I went to bed.

I was not told *why* I needed to go to the hospital or *what* the doctor who changed my prescription might be concerned about.

I wasn't a big fan of being ordered to do something by an authority figure *without* an explanation. In my way of thinking, that had ended when I was discharged from the U.S. Army in June 1971.

On that fateful day of April 12th, after getting out of bed, I slipped on a pair of shorts and a t-shirt. I walked slowly into the kitchen. I braced myself on one section of the kitchen counter, and I waited that way, catching my breath, before I tried to cook breakfast for myself.

Waking up was sometimes difficult for me from the lingering effects of the meds I took for my depression. When I lacked enough sleep, it made waking up that much worse. During the night of April 11th, I had only awakened twice. All things considered, that was pretty good over the course of six hours. But getting back to sleep had been a big problem.

After I caught my breath, I started cooking breakfast. The smell of the sizzling bacon from the frying pan was intoxicating. The fresh-brewed Starbucks house blend tantalized my nostrils as it wafted up from my coffeemaker. At least my "bronchitis" had not affected my sense of smell.

As soon as the scrambled eggs cooking in real butter were done, I plated them, the bacon, and two pieces of buttered rye toast.

I sat down and thoroughly enjoyed my breakfast. It included two cups of hot coffee with half and half.

I got up and braced myself against my kitchen table. The lack of adequate oxygen to my lungs due to my "bronchitis" was making me light-headed. I made it to the kitchen sink with my dishes, set them in the sink and rinsed them off knowing that I would wash them later.

I prepared cat food for my four cats — Sugar, Max, Thelma and Louise. I carried their food onto the front porch on that pleasant early spring day, and they greeted me warmly there. The foursome eagerly went after their meal. I lingered a couple of minutes talking to them in a daily ritual that I loved.

I returned to the living room from outside and eased down onto my couch. I sat there feeling somewhat exhausted from that small amount of effort I had just exerted. I was in a bag!

Without warning, I coughed up **a crimson lunger!** It came so fast and hard that I only had time to get the palm of my left hand over my mouth with a couple of inches of space between my mouth and hand.

That cough hurt like hell! What hurt me worse was the sight of the **cherry-red bloody sputum** in the palm of my hand.

I froze my gaze in astonishment at the goo for more than a moment. I swallowed hard. I endured several aftershock coughs.

The fog in my brain was playing me. So was the lack of oxygen to my brain from the "bronchitis." I could not differentiate between the two.

I got to my feet slowly. I wobbled momentarily until I got enough oxygen intakes. I shuffled into the kitchen, grabbed a paper towel and put the bloody goo on it. I put the paper towel and its contents into the left pocket of my shorts. I also took several more paper towels and put them in the waist band of my shorts in case I blew out another lunger.

I needed medical attention quickly.

I made it back into my bedroom and managed to get shoes and socks on, coughing all the while. Then I got on my feet, steadied myself, and weaved toward the front door, staggering through a hallway and across the living room. It took me two minutes to traverse sixty feet.

*****

With persistence and patience, I made it outside and then braced myself on the front porch railing. My Toyota Tundra truck sat parked on the street in front of my house some fifty feet away. At that moment, it appeared to be a mile away since walking even a short distance took all I had.

Breathing through my mouth, I mustered up all the drive I could.

Moving in very short steps, I completed my walk to the driver's side of my truck. I caught my breath. I turned my head and I coughed but could not stop more **bloody sputum** from landing on the asphalt street after it left my open mouth.

I opened the door and slid into the driver's seat. I waited several minutes for my head to clear slightly. I coughed, coughed, and coughed with more **crimson bloody sputum** deposited into a paper towel.

It never occurred to me as I was sitting in the driver's seat to call for an ambulance, go to a neighbor's house and ask for a ride, or call someone to take me to the hospital. My only thought was to get medical help on my own. I was so used to relying on myself and myself only in all areas of my life.

Yet I was in no condition to drive. It was a very bad idea for me to get behind the wheel. Damn stupid in fact. But that's what I did.

To get medical help, I needed to start and complete a five-mile car ride successfully.

On this day in my condition, it might as well have been a hundred mile trip.

Fortunately, I didn't need a MapQuest or a Thomas Guide. I knew the way to the hospital having been there hundreds of times over the years.

On two occasions during the five-mile trip through heavy morning traffic, I had to pull to the side of the road to rid my lungs of **bloody sputum**. Energy, concentration and strength in general were in short supply.

While trying to ease back into the flow of traffic, I didn't see a car coming behind me and the driver had to lock up all four wheels to avoid hitting my rear bumper. When the driver caught up to me, he flipped me off. I weakly mouthed the words "My fault — I'm sorry..." to him.

Despite being a moving road hazard, I was not involved in any traffic altercations before I arrived at the hospital.

*****

I eased the Tundra into a parking space in the Emergency Room parking lot at Valleydale Hospital Medical Center. I got out of the truck without falling, even though I felt dizzy.

A couple of minutes later, I entered the ER waiting room. After leaning against one wall, I made it another thirty feet to the sign-in sheet in front of the window where a triage RN was sitting behind the glass. That person is the one who does an initial assessment of your condition.

At 8:40 am, I filled out the single page sheet and wrote **"BLOODY PHLEGM!"** on it.

She came into view and said, "How may I — oh, God..." The nurse stopped in mid-sentence when she saw the **bloody mess** in the paper towel I showed to her.

She opened the door and held onto my arm. "I coughed it up, ten minutes ago," I said.

The nurse helped me onto a gurney in an empty room. She said, "We'll have someone from admitting get your information in a little while. Whatever you do, **do not leave!** Do not leave unless a doctor tells you to!"

She hurried out of the room and stopped in front of the nurses' station in the ER. She talked to a man wearing green scrubs. As she talked to him, he turned his head and glanced at me.

The man hurried into my room. It was the first time I had ever met Dr. Christopher Kuhlman, one of the residents in the family practice rotation at VHMC. Thankfully, he would turn out to be *the* doctor I needed on that day.

At that point, **more bloody sputum** made its way up from my lungs. I knew that I looked like creamed chipped beef on toast (also known as s--t on a shingle). I tried to find a comfortable position on the gurney. No such luck.

Dr. Kuhlman handed me a tissue. He then spoke to me like a man with a lot on his mind.

He said, "I know that you are very ill. I have to treat a couple of patients ahead of you. I promise that I will find out what is wrong with you before I go home at 7:00 pm. Please be patient. Call for help if you feel that you need it. Whatever you do, **do not leave this facility**."

He put his hand on my shoulder for a moment. We made eye contact and then he hurried out of the exam room.

I saw Dr. Kuhlman reach the nurses' station, where he picked up a phone and made a call. I was tired of propping myself up on the gurney, and I got off my elbows and laid my head down.

*****

It wasn't long before a clerk from admitting came in to get my billing information. I was in the system so that made it easier on both her and me.

Breathing was so difficult for me that I couldn't speak in complete sentences. The clerk was patient and cordial while I gave her my information.

After she left, the icy cold chills started kicking in. There were no sheets or blankets in sight. I shook with clattering teeth. Actually, I had spasms from the chills and twitched uncontrollably.

I could have easily been mistaken for a law enforcement suspect being tasered by some cop.

A nurse saw me and zipped into the room. She started searching in a couple of cabinets. She said, "I'll get a couple of blankets out for you."

Luckily she was successful in her search. Those blankets were a welcome relief.

Then a "vampire" showed up (a phlebotomist who wanted a blood sample). How she got the needle in my arm with me shivering I still don't know, but she did.

The phlebotomist was joined by an RN who came in to take my vital signs. After taking my vitals, the RN then spent a few minutes with me.

She inquired, "How long has this been going on?"

"Sixteen days and nights." Cough, cough, and cough!

She told me, "You have a very good physician assigned to you. Hang in there. I know that's not much to offer right now but we have you on the radar."

The RN left the room for a minute, and then reappeared. She inserted an intravenous line into my arm and hung a bag of fluids on a pole.

She also put a nasal cannula on my head and turned open a valve so I could get more oxygen, which I needed badly. She returned to my area about every forty-five minutes to recheck vital signs and to look at me.

*****

I managed to doze between visits of the RN.

When I was awake, I wondered about the diagnosis of "bronchitis." It bugged me.

This scenario did not fit with past episodes of bronchitis in my life. My thoughts made it as far as realizing that something was really wrong. Then I'd fall back into a sleeping state.

I lost track of the time as I lay on the gurney. I was pretty sure that several hours had passed before Dr. Kuhlman returned to my room. I checked my watch. Actually, almost five hours had passed since I had arrived at the front desk of the ER.

Dr. Kuhlman said, "Mr. Folck, I'm going to devote my full attention to you now. A person will be here in a minute to transport you to radiology for a chest x-ray. We'll go from there."

*****

A few corridors later and a few turns along the way and I arrived in radiology in a wheelchair pushed by someone from the transportation department. The tech that x-rayed me had his hands full getting me to stand straight and not move. On the third try, he got a usable chest film.

As soon as the film was ready, the x-ray tech viewed it. He made a beeline to a phone and made a call. After that, he put the film in a large envelope and handed it to me. Then it was back in the wheelchair and back to the ER, thanks to the person from transportation who pushed me.

*****

As soon as I got back, Dr. Kuhlman dashed into my room. I handed him the x-ray. He took a quick, close look at my heart area on the film.

While glancing at the film, he blurted out, "There's something on your chest x-ray that shouldn't be there. And it doesn't look good from what I can see of it. We need to do a chest scan to try to determine what it is. Just stay in the wheelchair. You'll be out of here in a minute or two."

In my mind, the bottom had just fallen out. Yet I was too sick to get anxious at the news. I knew that I needed to call someone.

I maneuvered the wheelchair to the table alongside the gurney I had been on earlier. I picked up the phone and called my girlfriend, Rochelle Sharon Martenson, aka Shelley. She did not pick up, so I left a voice message. I had already told her that I was driving myself to the hospital.

I said, "It's me. They found something on a chest x-ray. Not sure what it is. Doesn't look good. Going in for a chest scan — cough, cough, cough." I ended the call.

Later I found out from Shelley that she had gone into an absolute panic when she heard my message. She ran into the office manager's office at the law firm where she worked and informed her that she had to leave due to a medical emergency — *mine*.

The first thoughts that entered Shelley's mind upon listening to my phone message had to do with me having lung cancer. Her mom had successfully fought cancer a few years back. Shelley didn't know what else to think, but she was petrified.

*****

I felt that I was very close to finding out what was wrong with me. It wouldn't be much longer. At least I would know more than I did.

What could it be?

A man from transportation wheeled me to the place where a tech performed a scan on my chest. The tech took his time and did a thorough job. As soon as he finished the scan, he was on the phone.

A couple of minutes later, he said, "We're sending you back to see the doctor. He needs to go over a couple of issues with you."

With that, I was wheeled back to my room. Dr. Kuhlman and a nurse helped me back onto the gurney. I coughed a couple of times. Once I caught my breath, the doctor began speaking.

With a very calm demeanor, Dr. Kuhlman said, "The tech saw a spot on your chest x-ray and determined what it was on the scan."

There was something fatalistic in Dr. Kuhlman's voice that made me too stunned to react. My intuition told me that I was going to receive bad news.

Chapter 2—December 2003

Why did I feel that my world was coming apart at the seams in December 2003?

For one thing, my job situation was not going well at the time. More scrutiny than ever before was directed at property claims reps like me.

A recently installed information technology system to reduce claims costs was in place at Farmers Insurance. In all ways, it was a "Big Brother" system. Any supervisor or manager in claims could review your work at any time. If you made any errors, you heard about it from someone higher up in the company.

Individual initiative in settling homeowner claims was gone. My co-workers and I had become robots.

Plus, every day, there was a memo about a new change to the system. It was daunting to keep up with the changes.

With the additional stress I felt, my work suffered. My concentration and attention to detail waned. I had to re-do so many claims because of my errors.

With so much pressure on claims costs, phone calls to claimants were more difficult. Many simply objected to settlement offers and were quite vocal about their displeasure. These changes raised my stress level even more.

Also, there were more requests for additional money after claimants "remembered" or "discovered" that additional items were taken. Claims had to be re-opened and recalculated and more money paid out.

From my work experience at Farmers, I knew that every year from Halloween until Easter of the following year the volume of claims increased. It was a seasonal blip.

At times, after hearing some of the bogus stories about theft losses around the holidays, I wanted to say to certain people, "I'm sorry but we don't finance Christmas." Instead, I bit my tongue.

Another stressor was that claims reps were expected to work off the clock without additional pay, especially when co-workers took end-of-year vacations or when we were short-handed.

The major stressor was that my job, as I knew it, was going away. In time, there would be no more office claims reps. Farmers wanted able-bodied claims reps only.

This was a major problem with the bilateral osteoarthritis in my knees. Working inside let me avoid excessive walking, squatting, getting down on all fours, and walking on worn, uneven roof surfaces.

Dr. Friedland, my orthopedic surgeon, and I had worked very hard since 1999 to lessen the discomfort I had from O.A. We tried everything, including injections of synthetic cartilage.

*****

December brought with it significant anniversary dates for me. Both of my marriages had ended in December. The anniversaries of my arrival to and return from Vietnam occurred in December.

Still, in 2003, Christmas came and went with no extra difficulties for me. I set my sights on the end of the year and hoped for a better 2004.

However, throughout December 2003, my psychiatric condition, Post-Traumatic Stress Disorder (PTSD), had been beating on me with all the additional work-related stress that was on my plate.

The PTSD stemmed from my service in Vietnam with Company B, 554th Engineer Battalion (Construction). I was a welder.

*****

Without fail in December 2003, my sleep was interrupted between 4:30 am and 5:30 am daily. You could set your watch to it or start your day with its arrival. It had been that way for decades.

Sometimes my sleep was only slightly interrupted, and I could easily go back to sleep. On other occasions, it brought with it a nightmare or a flashback to combat which sometimes left me too rattled to sleep anymore.

My sleep was torpedoed by "Five O'clock Charlie," early on the morning of December 27, 2003. It was a doozy. All hell broke loose in my bed at about four in the morning.

*****

The basis of the flashback began at 3:43 am on February 26, 1969 at Cu Chi base camp. Members of the 272nd North Vietnamese Army (NVA) Regiment and local Vietcong (VC) broached the perimeter by blowing up a main defensive bunker with a satchel charge.

After cutting the perimeter wire, they ran upright onto the base toting RPGs, satchel charges, AK-47s and other weapons.

When I awoke to incoming rockets and mortars, I scrambled to a bunker outside my hooch.

After about three minutes of rockets and mortars, a sergeant announced, "Gooks are inside the wire. This is a ground attack. Guys are getting ambushed. Get into your hooches and put on your s--t and get to the secondary bunker line!"

All of us did as told at light speed. It was all assholes and elbows as we slipped on our pants, jungle boots, flak jackets and steel pots (helmets). We all grabbed our weapons and ammunition.

A steady stream of soldiers hurried to the secondary defensive bunkers as the attack continued on a dry, clear night.

34

I made tracks with my friend James McDonald.

As we neared our bunker, I saw a Vietnamese attacker barefoot and wearing a "diaper" toting an RPG launcher in our motor pool. He was about fifty yards away.

I almost went after him, but decided to get to my bunker instead.

Our bunker was a large culvert half-pipe with one layer of sandbags on it and a short wall of sandbags across the front opening maybe three high.

A direct hit on top of the bunker from an incoming 122 mm rocket would have killed us.

The secondary bunkers were about one hundred yards behind the main bunker line.

McDonald and I stayed, pinned down, in that bunker for the next two-and-a-half hours. All around us, a loud, raging battle ensued right before our eyes.

We heard AK-47 fire, small arms fire, machine gun fire, grenades exploding, exploding mortar rounds, some very large explosions and more.

A helicopter refuel depot and a re-arm area, with ammunition for Cobra gunships, was fifty yards behind the main bunkers.

A lucky enemy mortar round from the Cu Chi village landed in the re-arm point, and it exploded starting a massive, spectacular chain reaction. The initial explosion was the loudest explosion I have ever heard.

Decades later, I was diagnosed by the Department of Veterans Affairs of having a 20% bi-lateral hearing loss from that attack — mostly because of the re-arm point going up.

It took eight hours for the re-arm point to stop burning. In the meantime, stray rounds were flying randomly into the air in all directions. If any of us in those bunkers had ventured outside, there would have been a high likelihood that we would have been hit by exploding U.S. rounds.

At about 4:30 am an Air Force C-47 Spooky gunship appeared overhead and sprayed the ground between the secondary bunker line and the main bunkers and the area between the main bunkers and the wire with 20mm rounds from a mini-gun cannon on the aircraft. It seemed like the firing lasted an hour.

Every fifth round from the mini-gun was a tracer shell, meaning that the bullet glowed red as it went through the air. We saw red tracer shells **bouncing** off the earth around us.

All we could hear was the **growl** of the mini-gun spitting out rounds. That sound was deafening.

Dawn came and brought with it the images of dead enemy combatants and Army Chinook helicopters that had been satchel charged and burned into heaps of melted metal.

On the entire basecamp, fourteen U.S. soldiers were killed and twenty-eight were wounded. Thirty-one NVA soldiers were killed (by body count) and eight POWs were captured. Nine Chinook helicopters were destroyed and two were damaged.

Let me tell you, it was damn awful.

*****

My December 27, 2003 sleep interruption manifested itself as a flashback to combat of that February 1969 attack.[vi]

During the flashback, an imaginary group of North Vietnamese/Vietcong attackers in shiny black pajama pants toting AK-47s, RPGs, and satchel charges would enter my night time thoughts. They always screamed and were very, very angry at me. The nightmares always seemed so vivid and they haunted me. They seemed to be in Dolby sound.

*****

I remember striking out at my imaginary attackers on that December 27th morning with my flailing legs and feet using turbocharged leg kicks.

The kicking was so violent that it woke me up and made me sit straight up in bed.

At that time, my legs looked like they belonged to an NFL lineman. They were very large and heavily muscled. They had been like that since I was sixteen years old.

Once I woke up, I could see that my feet were entangled in my bed sheet and blanket. I finally managed to untangle them and lay back down. Fortunately, I was able to go back into a light sleep.

My girlfriend, Shelley, was in bed with me. I kicked her hard several times causing bruises to her legs.

Even though I was taking meds for my PTSD, my nighttime flashbacks were out of control. I've learned that sleep difficulties are common for people with PTSD, especially Vietnam combat vets.

When I woke up for good from the flashback that December morning, I was groggy from the effects of the meds I took for the PTSD. It took a moment or two for my head to clear.

I swung my legs off the bed and put my feet on the floor. My right knee was swollen and painful. It looked like a softball had been stuffed inside it. It hurt like hell.

It was then that I figured out that my knee bone was connected to my PTSD bone in a metaphorical sense.

I made it through the day, limping.

*****

Finally, night came. I crawled into bed. Once again I was fortunate to have my girlfriend Shelley spending the night.

Early in the morning of December 28, 2003, I had a recurring flashback. It was just as bad as it had been the night before. It was an identical nightmare.

The same imaginary attackers with their AK-47s and RPGs and satchel charges were in my head. They were yelling at me and they were trying to kill me.

Eventually, I woke up for good and put my feet on the floor. I noticed that my right knee was even more swollen than it had been when I had gone to bed.

I had kicked like a wild man trying to fend off the attackers in my flashback. Shelley had endured more kicks.

*****

According to the National Center for PTSD, Post-Traumatic Stress Disorder or PTSD is a psychiatric disorder.[vii] It may occur after one experiences or sees military combat, natural disasters, terrorist incidents, serious accidents, or violent personal assaults like rape. A majority of survivors of such trauma return to normal over time. Some people manifest stress reactions that do not go away on their own, or may even get worse over time. These persons may develop PTSD. People with PTSD often re-live the experience through nightmares or flashbacks, have diffficulty sleeping, and feel detached or estranged, and these symptoms can be severe enough and last long enough to significantly impair the person's daily life.

PTSD causes biological changes and psychological symptoms.

PTSD dates back to written records in ancient times, and there is clear documentation in the historical medical literature starting with the Civil War.

Psychophysiological alterations linked to PTSD include hyper-arousal of the sympathetic nervous system, increased sensitivity of the startle reflex, and sleep abnormalities.

PTSD also significantly impacts psychological functioning, independent of concurrent conditions of people in their daily lives. Vietnam veterans with PTSD were found to have profound and pervasive problems with family and in other interpersonal relationships, problems with employment, and involvement with the criminal justice system.

A litany of physical symptoms is tied to patients with PTSD including headaches, gastrointestinal complaints, immune system problems, dizziness, chest pain, and discomfort in other parts of the body. Often, medical doctors treat the symptoms without being aware that they stem from PTSD.

PTSD is treated by psychotherapy (talk therapy) and drug therapy. There is no definitive treatment, but some treatments appear to be quite promising — especially cognitive-behavioral therapy, and group therapy.

*****

I was formally diagnosed with "survivor's guilt" PTSD in 1993. I came home and almost 60,000 Americans in uniform did not. I lost two people over there who were important in my life. I felt guilt over the deaths of Clyde W. Saunders and Gerould M. Rumble, III.

After being diagnosed, I took old-style antidepressants like Desipramine and Imipramine to ease my symptoms. They took forever to start working, and these drugs had several unpleasant side effects, mainly a very dry mouth when speaking.

I also contended with panic attacks. I was given Klonopin for the panic attacks, which left me in a zombie-like state. I soon got off the Klonopin.

I participated in individual and group therapy at the Sepulveda Vet Center on the grounds of the Sepulveda V.A. Medical Center for more than nine years with occasional follow-ups.

I learned many techniques in therapy to cope with my PTSD. I had the benefit of some very caring people, unlike any I have met before or after. They helped me enormously.

In 2000, or 2001, I switched to a new antidepressant — venlafaxine or Effexor. It was a great antidepressant for the symptoms I had.

*****

I made an appointment to see Dr. William Rumack at the Orthopedic Medical Center in Reseda, California.

When I saw Dr. Rumack, he tapped my badly swollen right knee with a large volume hypodermic syringe and needle. He drained off 120 ccs of knee joint fluid.

An x-ray was also taken.

Dr. Rumack was incredulous that I had done so much damage to my knee from kicking my legs in bed.

At the end of the appointment, I was given home healthcare instructions to prevent further damage.

A few days later, I saw Dr. Jerome Friedland at Orthopedic Medical Center. He shook his head when I told him about the flashbacks causing my knee damage.

He tapped and drained my knee for another 90 ccs of fluid.

He told me that it was obvious that I had torn the medial meniscus in my right knee. This was on top of the osteoarthritis and my job stress.

Dr. Friedland gave me a prescription for pain meds and told me to stay off of my knee as much as possible. "Ice, ice, and more ice," he said.

I surmised that the buildup of work stress over the previous two months, plus knowing that I was about to lose my job, had caused me to erupt, mentally, in the middle of the night.

When you have PTSD, the stress has a number of ways that it can come out. In my case, it caused me to injure my knee. As far as PTSD goes, stress is stress. It does not differentiate among all the stressors you may have.

*****

Since July 1993, I have been the beneficiary of excellent psychiatric care from the Sepulveda V.A. Medical Center. My care has been world class.

Psychiatric residents from the UCLA School of Medicine see patients there on a regular basis. They have consulting psychiatrists available who are very experienced treating returning vets with PTSD. Many of the residents who treated me over the years have gone on to become successful psychiatrists in private practice.

For me, there was and still is no stigma attached to me requiring psychiatric care. I can't adequately describe nor detail how much good help I have received at that facility over the years.

*****

I went to see my psychiatric resident at the V.A. Medical Center in Sepulveda, California. Speaking slowly, I explained to him what had happened. He shook his head as he listened to my description of the events that transpired in my bedroom.

He advised me about my med dosage to ease the symptoms of my PTSD.

Even so, the doctor and I were concerned that this might be the start of increased activity with my PTSD. Neither of us looked forward to that prospect. Most of the time, it was difficult enough for me during that period.

One thing that the doctor was sure of, given how significant this episode appeared to be, was that I needed a sleep study. He wanted to capture my nightmare in full bloom in a controlled clinical setting.

He gave me a referral to the V.A. Wadsworth facility in West Los Angeles. He wanted me to be tested there for sleep apnea.

Like someone who had learned to cope with diabetes or some other chronic day-to-day illness, I had developed a set of coping skills for the symptoms of PTSD. Thank God I had done that.

When the symptoms were not debilitating, I went with the flow and got on with my life. When the symptoms were beating on me, I dug into my bag of coping tricks.

Plainly and simply, when my brain was in gear, I was a problem solver, not a whiner. My choice would have been to use my problem-solving abilities on other issues besides my knee dilemma and my PTSD, which had ramped up. However, those were among the crucial issues I was dealing with.

*****

I returned to work but was very uncomfortable both physically and mentally. I felt like there was a dark cloud hanging over my head about the longevity of my job.

On January 15, 2004, I received some bad news.

Nancy Vasquez, my Branch Claims Manager, called me into her office. Her dad had PTSD from his service in Vietnam and she empathized with me. Nancy had overlooked flaws in my performance.

Nancy told me that she was transferring to become the branch claims manager for a Farmers office in San Bernardino. In other words, my "protector" in the Calabasas office was leaving.

She told me, "There will be a new branch claims manager here after lunch. I'm not sure that you will 'fit in' with the new regime and his physical expectations."

I got up from the chair in front of her desk. We hugged. She kissed me on the cheek. I said, "I'll miss you."

I left the claims office and went to Van Nuys where I filed a claim for state disability. I was on the clock to receive disability payments. At the same time, I took a leave of absence under the Family Medical Leave Act. This meant that my job would be kept open, legally, until July 15, 2004.

Little did I know what would transpire in the coming days, weeks and months. Without giving anything away, July 15, 2004 would come and go as a blur. But that is for a later discussion.

*****

Several months passed.

I complied with Dr. Friedland's orders to stay off my right knee as much as possible. Yes, I really did need to be on state disability.

Dr. Friedland wanted to avoid another arthroscopic surgery on my right knee because I was running out of healthy cartilage in that knee. He prescribed a regimen of physical therapy, which I followed to the letter. I missed my regular physical activities, though, which included walking and riding my bike.

As you might expect with me getting less exercise than usual, my depression headed south. I consulted with my psychiatric resident at the V.A. We decided not to increase the dosage of my antidepressants.

By the latter part of March 2004, my right knee had only improved slightly. It wasn't responding to the physical therapy. It cried out for surgical intervention. Dr. Friedland and I made the decision that I needed arthroscopic surgery on my knee. His office nurse put me on the surgery schedule for April 9th.

It never occurred to me that a new portfolio of medical problems was ahead of me.

Chapter 3—The ER and Other Things

Have you ever heard the expression "the calm before the storm"?

March 27, 2004 turned out to be the kind of day realtors long for when showing properties. There was plenty of sunshine, mild temperatures and almost no wind.

I felt upbeat as I got my day started. I longed to be outside on that Saturday. I wanted my good mood to last.

I made up my mind to walk at Malibu Creek State Park in Calabasas. Its breathtaking open-spaces and outdoor scenery first lured me there years ago.

The Park contains a year-round stream fed by local "mountain" run-off, some gentle, rolling hills, a small dam that forms Freedom Lake (it's more like a pond), and numerous great hiking trails. There is a back part of the Park where water flows into the lake that has a great arch in a rock formation.

For decades, Malibu Creek State Park was used for outdoor movie and TV shoots. In fact, it is still used for location shoots today. ***Planet of the Apes, Windtalkers, Butch Cassidy and the Sundance Kid,* and *M.A.S.H.* (film and TV series)** are just some examples of film and television uses of the Park. One part of the Park still contains a jeep and an ambulance from the *M.A.S.H.* TV series.

You can work up a good appetite walking/hiking there. You also need to have water with you if you go.

*****

My daughter Melinda, my grandson Elijah and my granddaughter Jenasis arrived at my house to walk with me.

We piled in to Melinda's Ford van and drove to the Park.

Elijah was a toddler and Jenasis was four-and-a-half years old. I was so looking forward to a carefree day and a chance to be "Grampa."

Once at the Park, we enjoyed the singing birds, the gentle breeze that had picked up, and each other's company.

During that trip, I showed Jenasis and Elijah how to skip small flat rocks across still water in the creek. They loved it.

*****

After several hours in the Park, Elijah was too tired to continue. He had walked several miles and was out of energy

We made it back to Melinda's van as I carried Elijah on my shoulders. Jenasis wanted to ride on my shoulders, too. I begged off, telling her that I only had one pair of shoulders.

As I got in the van, I noticed that my right knee was painful and swollen. All the walking, plus carrying Elijah on my shoulders, had taken a toll on it.

I paid little attention to the discomfort. I had just enjoyed a lovely day with my family in a very beautiful and special place.

We stopped on the way home and I treated all of us to a very tasty fast food lunch after exerting so much energy. We kidded around and laughed inside the restaurant.

When we got back to my house, Melinda and the kids said their good-byes to me and they drove home.

I took an afternoon nap once I got inside.

After waking up, I watched a couple of favorite shows on the boob tube as I ate dinner.

During the night, a reminder of my mortality was building a case against my remaining a living, breathing human being.

Exactly when the campaign to do me in began, no one knows for sure. After the problem was discovered, sharp medical minds could not pin down a specific time or date for the start of it all. But that day, it was first brought to my awareness.

At 2:00 am on Sunday March 28, 2004, I awoke with a minor fever. I took my temperature and the thermometer read **100.5**.

I took two regular Tylenol for relief and then I crawled back into bed. The Tylenol seemed to do its job. I managed to fall back to sleep for five more hours.

I awoke sometime after dawn feeling feverish again. I checked my temperature one more time. The thermometer reading was 100.5 degrees Fahrenheit.

My fever was not debilitating. I went about my daily activities. I noticed that **my fever was intermittent** throughout the day.

Later that Sunday, I placed a call to Dr. Friedland. About fifteen minutes later, he called back.

I told him about my knee and my intermittent fever. I specifically said, **"Intermittent** fever."

He said, "You might have an infected knee."

He told me to go to the Emergency Room at Valleydale Hospital Medical Center in Valleydale. His instructions to me were to tell the doctor assigned to me to tap and drain my knee of excess fluid and to do a fluid culture of my knee joint fluid for any possible infection.

Friedland *never* mentioned that I should get a blood culture.

My girlfriend Shelley drove me to the ER at VHMC. Dr. Edward Nathan Morton was assigned my case.

I gave Morton a detailed explanation of the problems with my knee and what Dr. Friedland wanted him to do.

Morton tapped and drained my knee. He kept some of the fluid for a lab culture.

While he was still in the treatment room with me, he said, "I think that it is probably a good idea to do a blood culture." I agreed with him and a blood draw was ordered.

A phlebotomist drew blood on me.

I was told that I would be notified of the results of the blood culture by the hospital. As far as the results of the knee joint fluid culture, those would come from Dr. Friedland.

After that, I signed some papers, took my discharge instructions and left the Emergency Room.

I was not given any antibiotic. I was told to take Tylenol if the fever persisted.

It seemed like a very routine visit to the ER.

Once we were back at my place, I reassured Shelley that I was ok by telling her what had transpired regarding my visit to the ER.

*****

For the rest of that day and into the night, my knee was giving me fits. The pain continued unabated, the swelling was dramatic, and I did not have anything close to a full range-of-motion. I was anxious to see Dr. Friedland for his assessment of my knee. He had superb skills as far as diagnosing orthopedic issues.

I was able to get in to see Dr. Friedland that Monday, March 29, 2004. During that mid-morning office visit, I informed Dr. Friedland, and he saw firsthand, that my right knee was hardly bending at all.

He told me, "David, without the benefit of an MRI, I think that you aggravated your knee when you walked with your family and that some debris is in your knee cavity. It broke off due to the underlying osteoarthritis and is locking up your knee. This is on top of the torn medial meniscus. We need to go ahead and scope your knee," he said.

"What the hell. What's one more arthroscopy when you've been a frequent flyer," I mumbled.

"Even though Dr. Morton did a **fluid culture**, I want to do another one. **You can't be too careful when it comes to a possible infection, you know.**"

He then tapped and drained 100 ccs of fluid out of my right knee. I had really messed up big time by taking that walk with my family. He kept enough of the fluid for a culture.

Then I **coughed** in his exam room.

Dr. Friedland said, "I think you need to get someone to look at your cough. I don't want you going to surgery if you're having a respiratory problem."

I said, "I feel like crap."

He said, "Don't be afraid to ask for something good to treat it."

*****

Around 2:00 am the next morning, I woke up with a pain in my left wrist.

To compensate for my bad right knee, I had been bracing myself upon rising from a sitting position off of my living room couch using my left hand

and wrist. The more times that I got to my feet, the more times I put pressure on it.

My wrist was so sore by then that I felt I'd better have someone at the Emergency Room take a look at it.

I drove to the ER at Valleydale Hospital and signed in to triage at 3:09 am.

A physician's assistant named William Kent was assigned to me. He examined my wrist, ordered an x-ray and then went over the results with me.

During the initial intake with him, I mentioned that I had been to the ER there at Valleydale on the 28th of March for my right knee and a fever. **I told him that a blood draw was taken at that time for a culture as well as a fluid culture for my knee.**

William Kent *never* checked the hospital system to determine what the results were from the blood culture or the knee joint fluid culture. He never ordered my chart from the records department.

He gave me a prescription for pain meds, a muscle relaxer for my wrist, and a wrist brace to wear during the day. I was instructed to avoid using my wrist as much as possible.

I went home while it was still dark outside.

I went back to bed thinking that things would start improving for me.

*****

I woke up later that same morning of March 30 for the first time with the worst chills I could ever remember. My teeth clanked and I endured full body spasms from the chills.

I rode out the chills, got up with my wheezing cough, and had some hot chocolate. At that moment, I was grateful for microwave ovens and instant hot chocolate mix.

I continued to cough but I now had a noticeable wheeze. The **fever** remained **intermittent**.

I made an appointment that Tuesday to see Dr. Raymond Andrews, an internist who I had seen before for erectile dysfunction. His office was in Canoga Park, California, which was very close to my home.

My expectation of Dr. Andrews was that he was an experienced physician who could treat what ailed me.

Later that day (March 30) at his office, he took my vital signs, looked in my ears, checked my throat and used a stethoscope while I breathed. **Raymond Andrews also listened to my heart**.

I informed Dr. Andrews that I had been feverish between 100 degrees Fahrenheit and 101 degrees Fahrenheit since the early morning of March 28th. Furthermore, I told him that the cough I presented began on the 29th.

I specifically told him that my **fever** was **"intermittent."**

I did not mention that I had been to the Emergency Room at Valleydale Hospital Medical Center on March 28th. He did not ask if I had spoken to another doctor about my condition.

He thought for a moment and said, "I'm going to treat you for **bronchitis**."

A man of few words, Dr. Andrews also reflected that in his patients' records. His entries were very short.

He prescribed **Biaxcin**. I scheduled a follow-up visit and then left his office to fill the prescription. I also had prescriptions for a chest x-ray and a blood draw.

I felt crappy so I simply ignored his request to get the chest x-ray and have a blood draw done.

That was not at all like me. I didn't have a history of ignoring a doctor's orders. Until that day, I was a very compliant patient as far as following doctors' orders.

April 6th arrived with a thud. I was still going downhill with my "bronchitis" and a fever and chills. I recorded new highs in my temperature every day.

I had a follow-up appointment with Dr. Andrews that morning at 9:00 am. Shelley drove me to his office.

When I saw him, he took vital signs, looked at my throat, checked my ears, listened to my chest and **listened to my heart**.

I told him, "My fever is worse."

"One oh two point nine...?" he queried with a skeptical look on his face.

"Yes. It has been that high twice in the last few days."

He gave me an old-fashioned mercury thermometer, which I put under my tongue. A couple of minutes later, he removed it and checked the reading.

He noted, "It's about a hundred. And you still have bronchitis."

Dr. Andrews looked at me directly. "Are you sure it's been that high?"

"Yes."

"I'm not seeing that."

"I'm not any better. The stuff you gave me doesn't seem to be working too well."

After a pregnant pause, Dr. Andrews said, "I'm going to switch you to another antibiotic—**Augmentin**."

I didn't know Augmentin from augmentation.

He wrote out the prescription and handed it to me.

In a very serious voice, he queried, "Did you get that chest x-ray and blood draw I asked you to get last week?"

I slumped forward, bowed my head and shook it side to side indicating "no."

"I need you to get those things done today! Do you understand me?"

I nodded "yes."

"If you can't drive, can someone take you?"

"Yes, my girlfriend can take me."

"I'll see you back here in three days."

He handed me a new prescription for a chest x-ray and one for a blood draw.

Dr. Andrews never ordered a **blood culture and sensitivity** for me, just the blood draw.

In the doctor's waiting room, I told Shelley that we needed to make a few more stops in order to get further clarity about my condition.

*****

Shelley then drove me to a medical facility in Northridge where I got a chest x-ray.

After that, Shelley took me to a lab where a blood draw was done.

After I finished, Shelley gave me a ride to a pharmacy where I filled the prescription for Augmentin. She wanted us to go have lunch, but I felt too wiped out all things considered.

Once I got home, I headed for the couch.

At my request, Shelley called Dr. Andrews later in the day and left a voicemail message for him. She told him that I was so ill that I could barely speak and that I had very, very bad chills.

A little later, Dr. Andrews called me. He told me to return to the ER at VHMC to be seen there. He said that I should get a chest x-ray and a blood draw.

Once, again, at that point, Shelley stepped up to the plate for me and drove me to the ER at Valleydale Hospital.

*****

It was the early afternoon when I signed in at the VHMC Emergency Room.

Shelley was so worried about me that she endured an awful migraine that eventually caused her to vomit.

I was triaged at the walk-in entrance to the ER and put in a very small exam room. An RN came in, took my vital signs, and made a few notes about why I was there. I detailed everything from March 28th on and my current diagnosis of "bronchitis," plus treatment with Augmentin.

I emphasized that I was not getting any better and that my condition was getting worse. I hacked and wheezed a couple of times. I was sweating from the fever.

A few minutes later, Edward Nathan Morton, MD, the same doctor I had seen previously at the same ER, entered the small exam room I been assigned to. He was alone and asked what seemed to me to be some "**off the wall**" questions.

"What is your home phone number?"

"Eight one eight, xxx-xxxx."

"That's what it says on the sheet. Do you speak Spanish?"

I got the most puzzled look on my face.

"No."

"Is there anyone at your house who speaks Spanish?"

"No. I live alone. No one who comes to my house speaks Spanish. Why are you asking me these questions?"

"A clerk in the Emergency Room tried to reach you by telephone. According to her notes, which I have here, she reached someone who only spoke Spanish."

He nervously glanced at the information on the clipboard.

"The reason that she was calling was to give you the results of your blood culture. You have a blood *Staph.* infection. I see that Dr. Andrews prescribed Augmentin for you. **Augmentin will take care of any infection you have.**"

*****

During this visit, Edward Nathan Morton MD: listened to my lungs with a stethoscope; did not say anything further about the nature of my blood infection; did not say whether or not the infection would remain in my blood if the wrong antibiotic were prescribed; did not order an ultrasound of my chest area; did order a consult with a specialist; did not mention anything about possibly admitting me to the hospital for observation; did nothing to check to see if there was a change in my white blood cell count; did not tell me anything about the sensitivity of my blood infection to certain antibiotics, which was available on the hospital computer system; did not say anything about lab results on blue paper versus white paper; and he did not listen to my heart.

*****

Ron C. Fujita, MD entered the exam room as I sat on the edge of the bed. He was a resident in the family practice residency program at VHMC. As part of that program, Dr. Fujita had to spend a certain number of hours working in the Emergency Room.

Dr. Fujita gave me paperwork to sign and reminded me to follow up with Dr. Andrews. He did not give any indication that the follow-up was urgent nor did he indicate that I should call Dr. Andrews immediately.

Dr. Fujita barely spent two minutes with me from what I can remember. I have stood in line for fast food longer than he was in the exam room with me.

Dr. Fujita failed to do the same things that Dr. Morton failed to do and he had the same information about me that Dr. Morton did.

At that moment, I left the ER satisfied with the knowledge that I had the **correct antibiotic** for my "bronchitis." In reality, that was far from the truth about what was going on in my chest.

Shelley drove me home and I went to bed. That night, the fever and chills alternately hammered me, plus I had several coughing frenzies.

*****

I saw Dr. Andrews on the 9th of April as planned. He took vital signs, listened to my chest, **listened to my heart**, checked my ears and looked down my throat. I told him that the high fever persisted. He checked my temperature and it was only 101 degrees Fahrenheit.

He saw no need to make any changes.

He told me to come back on April 12th. He said nothing about my blood infection. Dr. Andrews did not inform me of the results of the chest x-ray he had ordered nor the results of the labs he had ordered. He didn't say anything about talking with Dr. Ron C. Fujita by phone.

*****

By Saturday, April 10, 2004, I was about to lose my mind from trying to cope with my "bronchitis." All of my symptoms were worsening.

The crisis crescendo in my body was building to an unbelievable climax.

The high fevers made me delirious. The Richter scale chills were awful.

Everything about my condition was manifested in my physical being. I looked like: forty miles of bad road; what the cat dragged in; or a walking corpse.

The bed sheets I slept on were permeated with perspiration day and night. My briefs and t-shirt would get wringing wet from the sweating.

Could I endure any more of this? Was I really just dreaming?

My girlfriend Shelley was with me on the evening of the 10th being her guardian angel self.

Although I wanted to speak to her, the chills were so bad that I couldn't talk. I couldn't open my mouth far enough, just enough to feel my upper and lower jaws bang against one another over and over.

My brain searched for solutions to my sleep problems. My past experiences with sleep deprivation were not good.

I thought that I had caught the all-time hellish case of bronchitis! Son-of-a-bitch, it was nasty or was it a dream?

Finally, I summoned up the brain power and logic to conclude that the Augmentin was not working.

Meanwhile, talking was very difficult — PERIOD. My breathing was shallow and labored, I was coughing, and then there were the chills. These all negatively impacted my ability to speak.

I asked Shelley to call Dr. Andrews.

She spoke to a person at his answering service. Shelley explained what was going on with me and that Dr. Andrews needed to call back.

*****

About thirty minutes later, the phone rang. It was Andrews.

"Dr. Andrews, I'm Dave Folck's girlfriend. He is not doing well. It's hard for him to talk, to breathe, and he can't sleep."

Dr. Andrews responded to her but I did not hear what he said.

Shelley tried once again to give Dr. Andrews the 4-1-1 on my condition. She talked and talked and talked.

In a failing voice, I said, "Honey, let me talk to him."

She handed me the phone.

I coughed a couple of times before I spoke into the receiver.

In the strongest voice I could muster, I asked, "What is the strongest antibiotic you can give me for my bronchitis?"

"That would be **Levaquin**."

Levaquin is also known as Oxacillin.

"Good. That's what I want! **Augmentin isn't working**."

Then I had a coughing fit. I was pretty sure that I could have launched a lung at that point.

"I'll give you a prescription for Levaquin but you need to get yourself to a hospital."

"Why??? They haven't done a thing for me! All they did was prescribe Tylenol!"

He never responded.

58

I handed the phone back to Shelley and she gave him the number of a pharmacy to call. They ended the call while I had another coughing fit.

I was so bleeping tired of asking for help from medical personnel and not having them come through for me. I had asked for help for two weeks without getting what I needed.

Why couldn't anyone see what was going on? Did this fit the pattern for "bronchitis"?

It seemed that Dr. Andrews was only chipping away at the problem I had presented to him. He didn't seem to understand how ill I was. I was quite exasperated and frustrated by the lack of progress from his treatment plan.

I thought to myself, "If what I have is, in fact, bronchitis, there is a cure for it."

*****

Shelley drove to the Sav-On pharmacy in Northridge and picked up the prescription for Levaquin. I took one of the tablets as soon as she got back with them. Feeling as lousy as I did, I gathered up enough energy to give her a hug. I thanked her big time for getting the Levaquin. She had really saved the day for me since I was in no condition to drive.

Shelley stayed with me and watched over me. She did her level best to make me comfortable. Eventually, I went to bed several hours after taking the first dose of Levaquin.

*****

That night, I only woke up once. While I was awake, I took the second dose of Levaquin. I knew that I needed to have an elevated level of the medication in order to have a shot at getting better.

My PTSD was at bay that night. 5 O'clock Charlie took the morning off. It was a blessing.

The chills and fever were minor league that night.

*****

Easter Sunday of 2004 fell on April 11th.

When I got up that morning, **I noticed that both of my forearms had scratches that were scabbed over. The scratches had occurred while I was tending to the rose bushes on the property where I lived. I probably got them about the 25th of March.**

I felt well enough that Sunday to go to a holiday dinner at Marie Callender's restaurant in Northridge with Shelley and her family. That's not to say or imply that I was making a miraculous recovery from "bronchitis." I coughed frequently and the coughing was painful. I did feel a sense of optimism that day, but I am optimistic by nature.

In my mind, the Levaquin was working. Finally, Dr. Andrews had hit the nail on the head with a treatment for me.

My knee problems were not so troubling at that time. Having been off my feet so much in the preceding days had been a big help to them.

At bedtime I looked forward to getting over my "bronchitis" and getting my life back within a few days on the new antibiotic. I had had enough of being ill. I felt that I could put the last two weeks behind me very quickly. I fell asleep quickly.

Chapter 4—Later on April 12th, 2004

How would you feel if you experienced more drama in one day than you had ever felt cumulatively in your entire life?

*****

Dr. Kuhlman looked me right in the eyes, then said, **"You have infectious bacterial endocarditis from a** *Staphylococcus aureus* **blood infection."**

I bowed my head and gently shook it back and forth. I raised my head from my chest and opened my eyes.

In summary, Dr. Kuhlman told me that: My heart had an infection growing around it; it had been growing over time due to the blood *Staph.* infection; I had a vegetative growth on my heart valve; and I had triple bacterial pneumonia.

My chest heaved as much as it could as I tried to get the deepest breath that I was able to muster.

Dr. Kuhlman added, "I'm issuing an order to have you admitted to the hospital immediately to treat the infection. You're going to be here for several days or longer."

The ER doctor put his right hand on my left shoulder. "We know exactly what we're dealing with, Mr. Folck. There is no mystery anymore. As you have probably figured out by now, you are gravely ill from the infection. We will do whatever we need to do to help you through this. We won't know the extent of all that may be wrong with you until we do further tests. A tech will perform an echocardiogram on you to check all of your heart functions. Several doctors and medical people from the hospital will talk to you upstairs."

I closed my eyes for a moment. Then I regained whatever composure I had left.

I thanked Dr. Kuhlman for keeping his promise to find out what was wrong with me before his shift ended. We shook hands and he left the room. It was late in the afternoon. His shift was almost over.

My 24/7 shift of the fight of my life was just beginning.

*****

At least this ER doctor correctly diagnosed my medical condition. I can't say the same for two other Emergency Room doctors I had seen, especially one in particular.

My next thought was "**Bronchitis my ass!**"

A heart infection growing in size for two to three weeks. Triple pneumonia. What the hell went wrong? How did this happen?

Someone had been feeding me steer manure!

Emotionally, I was at once even more depressed than I had been. Then my mood changed. It took about twenty minutes for the transition. Then I was raging inside with anger knowing what infirmities I had. Yet I had no energy to manifest my anger on the outside.

The thoughts continued. Heart infection? Does this mean a heart attack might occur? How do you treat this? What happens next? What else could be wrong? Has any damage been done to my heart? My lungs? My brain? Hell, my brain can't be damaged any more than it is.

The fog from depression in my brain and the lack of adequate oxygen torpedoed my thoughts pretty quickly. My mind felt as if it were in a vegetative state. As I would later learn, one part of my body *was* in a vegetative state.

As was usually the case, I "steeled up" for whatever might be ahead when trouble came calling. I could fall apart later.

My chills, teeth clanking, shaking, twitching, spasming, and shivering continued.

*****

How the bacteria got into my bloodstream might have happened like this…

A simple sneeze against my forearm as I tried to block the nasal spray of the sneeze may have transferred bacteria from inside my nose onto my skin. After that, a scratch from a rose thorn that drew blood could have allowed the bacteria into my blood.

I did not contract *Staphylococcus aureus* in a hospital setting. You would think that the discovery of those bacteria in my body in late March 2004 would have set off alarm bells to trained physicians and other hospital personnel in the ER. However, that was not the case.

*****

A man from the transportation department of the hospital wheeled me from the ER to a waiting elevator, then to my room.

Once I was settled, I made a series of distasteful phone calls.

Shelley was called first. She said that she was on her way. I told her that I would fill her in when she got to my room.

My son Darrell was next. I left a message on his voicemail to call me at VHMC.

My daughter Melinda was third. The conversation with her was very emotional as I described my plight. I told her that it all went downhill after we had walked at Malibu Creek State Park with her kids.

She was completely overwhelmed and broke into tears for several minutes. I have never heard her cry that hard.

She asked, "How did this happen? Except for your appendix, you've never been really sick from anything during my life! What happened?!"

"I don't know how the infection got into my blood stream; I don't know, honey..."

"Don't die on me — I need you in my life for a long time," Melinda said.

We said our good-byes after a few minutes.

Then I made the hardest phone call of all to my brother.

"Hello, this is Forrest."

"Hi."

"You don't sound good."

"I've been admitted to Valleydale Hospital with a heart valve infection and triple pneumonia."

Obviously shocked at the news he said, "What?!!!"

"I got the news about an hour ago from an ER doc."

"What happened?"

I gave him a blow-by-blow.

We chatted for a few more minutes. I asked Forrest to tell his son and daughter that I was in the hospital. I told him that I would call back when I knew more.

*****

This is the stuff that **just crushes family members**. Yet the guilty just try to play everything down. They talk in reserved voices and look for excuses.

Malpractice hurts the injured patient and it wreaks havoc on that person's family. And the potential wrongdoers don't give a damn unless you sue their asses and then they run for cover.

*****

Matthew Schwinger, MD came into my room as if he didn't want to bother me but he had to.

We shook hands.

Dr. Schwinger indicated that I needed various tests and scans of my heart in order to get a comprehensive picture of what I was facing.

He informed me that in twenty-four hours, he could tell me the extent of the damage to my heart and my prognosis.

He advised me, "You have a **one centimeter vegetative growth** on your heart valve that is a very serious condition."

He held my hands as he looked at my fingers and fingernails.

Dr. Schwinger took his stethoscope from around his neck and put the ends in his ears. He listened to my breathing after placing the stethoscope on my middle back.

"Please take some normal breaths."

So I did.

Then he listened to my heart for the **distinctive and tell-tale murmur** of an aortic heart valve that had gone bad.

It is called a *diastolic* murmur. It has a sound all unto its own.

Only I didn't know he was listening to a heart murmur.

"You're going to be here for a while," he said.

We chitchatted for another minute and then he left.

*****

Around this time, Shelley came into my room, walked up alongside me, and hugged me the best that she could.

Her face told the tale. She looked very fearful.

I found the words to tell Shelley what had been discovered about my condition so far. It didn't take long for her to lose it.

She bawled for five minutes. Then she started to pull it together.

A few years earlier, Shelley had lost her ex-husband to a fatal heart attack. He and I were about the same age and both of us were large, tall men. Unlike me, her ex had abused his body with his lack of physical exercise, drinking and smoking. He was in a bad way health-wise when he passed on.

*****

Next, two physicians entered my room while Shelley was still there. This was my first encounter with Mark Amico, MD, who was in charge of the family practice residency program at VHMC.

Dr. Amico was an internist. He was a physician at the Northridge Family Practice Medical Clinic as well.

He introduced himself and the other physician who was with him, Tigalat Shalita, MD, a resident in the family practice program.

Their small pen flashlights came out and they started giving me the once-over. Each of them listened to my chest and breathing for several minutes. After that, they looked at each other.

Dr. Amico put his stethoscope directly over my heart on my chest and listened for several minutes. He listened and listened and listened.

He asked Dr. Shalita to listen to my **heart murmur**.

I responded with "Heart murmur? I don't have a heart murmur."

Dr. Amico said, "Yes, you do. I can hear it very clearly. This one has a distinctive sound."

I turned to Shelley and said, "I can't believe it."

She covered her mouth and nose with her hands. Then she cried a little more.

Dr. Shalita took his turn with his stethoscope. After about a minute, he pulled it off my chest.

I said, "Dr. Amico, what… what is the significance of my heart murmur?"

"Your aortic valve, the one that pumps blood through the aorta, is not closing all the way like it is supposed to. So the blood regurgitates causing the murmur sound. It's because it was damaged by the infection you have that got into your bloodstream."

"You mean that the infection ate part of my valve?!"

"That seems to be the most likely scenario."

"Jesus!!…"

Ever the one to summarize a situation, I gave him the abridged version of what had happened, including who did and didn't do what, when, why and how, and how slowly/quickly.

As Dr. Amico looked me right in the eye, he said, "This **never** should have happened to you. Because you were not notified in a timely manner and then not treated with the correct antibiotic, the infection in your blood grew in a cluster on your aortic valve. It grew unabated and wrecked that valve. It also clustered in three areas of your lungs, giving you triple bacterial pneumonia."

67

Shelley shook her head.

I felt powerless and helpless as I swallowed hard.

Dr. Amico added, "Your heart valve is in a **vegetative state**. You may need surgery to replace that valve."

Then Dr. Amico directed my attention to my hands and especially my fingernails.

"You see the little red spots you have?"

"Yes."

"They're called splinter hemorrhages. They're a sign of the problem with your heart."

I looked more closely. They were everywhere on my fingers and hands. Dr. Shalita also looked at them.

The doctors left together. Shelley would be visiting with me for quite a while longer.

*****

A few moments later, Michael Soltero, MD, entered my room.

Dr. Soltero gave me three options for treating my condition. They were: one, do nothing and you will die in three to four days; two, clear up the infection and try to live with a heart that is not fully functional; and three, clear the infection, the pneumonia and surgically replace the bad aortic heart valve.

Almost immediately, I said, "I want to have the surgery."

"You have three choices for the type of heart valve you want. First, an artificial valve. Second, a "pig" valve. Third would be a human tissue valve."

"I don't have a clue."

Soltero gave some information about each option. At that point, I had questions.

"A human tissue valve will be the most resistant to infection, which is your biggest issue going into surgery. If you choose an artificial valve, there will be a 'touch and go' period to get rid of the infection. Also, you'll need to be on Coumadin for the rest of your life if you choose that option."

"Will I need Coumadin if I take the human tissue valve?"

"No. If you take the human tissue valve, you may need a replacement surgery in ten to fifteen years. Or it could last longer than that."

Or shorter, I thought.

I said, "Let's go for the human tissue valve."

"I'll schedule the surgery for one week from today on the morning of the 19th. Your valve will still be infected when we go in, but it's your lungs that we need to treat now so you can receive general anesthetic. We can't wait any longer than a week because there are risks for a stroke or a heart attack if we delay the surgery that long. We'll start you on **I V Levaquin**, which is the correct antibiotic for your condition."

"Are you sure...? I was told that I was on the right medication when Dr. Andrews put me on Levaquin."

"You were not given the correct type of Levaquin, Mr. Folck. Oral Levaquin is insufficient in your case. What happened to you **never** should have happened. It was right there to see."

With years of experience shining brightly as he spoke, Dr. Soltero said, "If other parts of your heart proximate to the aortic valve are really torn up, our only choice will be the mechanical/artificial valve. If so, that valve could get badly infected from the *Staph.* infection and it will be a real street fight to get rid of the infection. I'm hoping that we'll be ok on that, but a mechanical valve is a possibility."

He left and my room was an eerie looking place at that moment. The room was completely dark save for a little light from the bathroom. It was dark outside. The bathroom door was three-quarters closed.

Shelley got close to me and held my hand tightly. I didn't look at her because I knew that I would cry.

*****

Some time passed, and then a nurse came into the room and hung a bag containing Levaquin on my intravenous pole.

Shelley stayed. There was no doubt that she was very troubled by the news she heard.

When Shelley left, I called someone I knew who might have some insights into my situation. My first ex-wife, Wendy, had earned an M.S. in Nursing and also had a law degree. She was employed as a medical malpractice defense attorney. For part of her nursing career, she had been a coronary care unit supervisor.

I gave her the run-down on my situation.

Wendy said, "Someone is going to pay for this. Wow! How could they let this happen in this day and age?"

I asked Wendy about her experience at UCLA where she had her mitral heart valve replaced due to a congential defect. At that time, UCLA was considered "the place" to go for heart problems in Southern California.

Wendy spoke highly of the surgeon who had changed out the valve and about the level of care she received at UCLA. I thanked her for her input and said good-bye.

My son, Darrell, then age twenty-eight, was standing in the doorway to my hospital room. I motioned for him to come in.

Darrell was trying to tough it out. I had seen the look that he had on his face before.

"You got the joker, Pops."

70

My spirits picked up with this visit from Darrell and I gave him a synopsis of what I had learned.

Tearfully, he said, "I love you, Dad. I know that you are a very strong person. If there is a way to get through this, you'll figure it out."

"If all goes well in the next week, and I don't die of a stroke or a heart attack by then, he'll open me up. If it goes South, I don't want to live on any machines, ok? And tell 'em to bury me upside down so the world can kiss my ass. Your sister knows what I want in my coffin."

Then we got away from the reality of my situation and talked about some funny experiences we had had together. We were both laughing, even though it made me cough. I am always willing to laugh.

Finally, Darrell had to drive home to his place in Whittier so he left.

*****

I was finally alone with my thoughts. I was fifty-five years old and I needed a heart valve. And I wanted to kill someone about this!

I pondered whether I should have the surgery at VHMC, where part of this grand screw-up had originated. Or should I go somewhere else like UCLA Medical Center or Cedars-Sinai Medical Center?

While replacing a heart valve may not have been a surgery performed every day at VHMC, the information and body of knowledge of such a procedure was substantial there. I felt that the hospital had the necessary equipment and personnel to perform the surgery.

If I decided to go somewhere else, it would waste precious treatment time. I was also aware of Dr. Amico's advice not to move around too much.

"You need to stay in bed. Otherwise," he said, "you run the risk of having the infection break apart and migrate somewhere else in your body or brain, which could be fatal."

Enough said.

I felt that Dr. Soltero was a very experienced surgeon. He had been specific about things that only a hands-on surgeon would know. For this type of surgery, he was well-qualified. The supporting doctors also seemed very competent.

In addition, I sensed, from the moment I had arrived upstairs in my room, that the "fix was in," meaning that everyone who saw my chart knew what had happened and now they did not want to lose me. That's how the "fix was in." Another message that I got from my nurse and others was a similar refrain. In an exasperated voice, she said, "The complications that did in your heart valve **never** should have happened."

TRANSLATION: You have grounds for a malpractice case even if it is against my employer.

Meanwhile, I felt like a heart patient on some TV soap opera with the "Beep, beep, beep" of a monitor sounding in the background.

*****

Out of the blue, I remembered a Three Stooges short called *Men in Black*.

In that film, Larry, Moe and Curly were zany doctors in a hospital. They drove through the facility in little motorized cars, with Curly saying, "Wub wub wub wub wub wub wub!" The film was nominated for an Academy Award. It was hilarious!

Thank God that Moe Howard wasn't my surgeon!

*****

There was an ironic component to my situation. I was laid up in a hospital with a bacterial infection that went nuclear on my body, and there were people in hospitals all over the United States at the same time I was that could contract *Staphylococcus aureus* during their respective hospital stays since hospital acquired *Staph. Aureus* infections were so frequent.

*****

One of the last members of the hospital staff to enter my room that night was an infectious disease control specialist. She offered up that there was a possibility that I might have **tuberculosis**.

I exclaimed, "What?! Are you crazy?"

She said that they couldn't take any chances about TB since it was highly contagious.

For the next few days, I wore "protective" clothing so that the staff and other patients would not be at risk if I had TB.

The whole time that I wore the stuff, I thought of myself as "TB Dave."

Could it be true — a bad heart valve, triple pneumonia, and possibly TB? I seriously considered calling Shelley to see if she could bring me anything alcoholic to drink.

What would be next? What other possible complication could surface?

One of the thoughts that entered my head was "Would my penis fall off?"

*****

The next evening during my stay at VHMC, a nurse came into my room and saw Shelley without a mask over her face.

The nurse said, "Ma'am, you need to put a mask on over your face. The patient may have TB. It is transmitted in the air, in case you're not aware of it."

Shelley shot back with "Well, I don't think that my boyfriend has TB! If he does have it, I've already been exposed to it because I have been in this room before without a mask on! It pisses me off that people at this hospital blew the treatment of his infection... and now you're worried about TB?!"

You could hear the edge in her voice. She was "mama bear" at that moment.

My maternal grandfather, Clarence Lewis Melcher, died of TB in 1926. My mom was only five years old when he died. She told me about it when I was in my teens. It was the main reason she chose Nursing as her major at the University of Iowa. During and after her studies, my mother was much attuned to public health issues in nursing.

*****

The tests, blood draws for labs and so forth, the streams of medical personnel in my room, the screenings, and every other kind of interruption never ceased. It reminded me of my stay at UCLA as a boy when a doctor found the kidney infection that was giving me such trouble. None of it made me happy.

Intellectually, I knew that I needed to have all of it done. Nonetheless, I was sick of it after two days.

April 12, 2004 was the worst day of my life because of the news. It was also a great day because at last I knew what I was facing.

That is how I dealt with a day filled with more drama than I have ever had cumulatively in my whole life to date.

Chapter 5—*Staph. Aureus* and Bacterial Endocarditis

Staphylococcus aureus or *Staph. aureus,* according to *Wikipedia,* was first observed by surgeon Sir Alexander Ogsten in pus from surgical abscesses in 1880 in Scotland.[viii]

Staphylococcus aureus bacteria can transfer from person to person by simple contact. Transfer can also occur via contact to the human body with an item that has *Staphylococcus aureus* on it: a towel; an article of clothing; a bed sheet; a medical instrument; a syringe needle; mucus from a sneeze.

Common manifestations of *Staphylococcus aureus* are boils, pimples, impetigo, abscesses on the skin and other skin conditions. It is found in life-threatening diseases such as pneumonia, meningitis, toxic shock syndrome (TSS), osteomyelitis, endocarditis, bacteremia, sepsis and other medical conditions.

Staphylococcus aureus is commonly found among hair follicles in the nose, under one's arms, on the scalp and on other parts of the body where hair is present. To check a patient for *Staphylococcus aureus,* a swab from each nostril is taken. Or, if a doctor suspects that it is causing a blood infection, a blood draw is taken for a culture.

The best defense against the bacterium is to shower or take a bath or shower daily, and wash your hair. Regular hand washing is also helpful. Changing bath linen and bed sheets and the towel you dry off with regularly is helpful to reduce the likelihood of contracting it.

Endocarditis is an inflammation of the inner layer of the heart, also known as the endocardium. The most commonly affected structures with endocarditis are the **heart valves**.

Bacterial endocarditis means that the inflammation is due to the effects of bacteria. Infectious bacterial endocarditis to a heart valve, which is what I had, works in a manner that I will now describe.

Since the valves of the heart do not receive a blood supply through capillaries and or blood vessels, defense mechanisms such as white blood cells are not present to fight an infection to a heart valve. So, if a bacterium establishes itself on a valve, the body cannot get rid of it without help (**a correct antibiotic**). If the heart valve becomes damaged in any way prior to the infection being present in the blood, even by the process of aging, the bacteria have an excellent chance to grow right on the valve in a damaged spot. A damaged spot could be a *minute* nick in the valve or a spot affected by long-term wear and tear. Since blood flows through the valve, it goes over the infection and can clot on the damaged, infected area. A deformed valve also presents opportunities for bacterial endocarditis.

An infection might enter your bloodstream via a minor cut or abrasion (*community acquired*) as can be the case with *Staphylococcus aureus*. Or it can come from a medical instrument like a hypodermic needle (*hospital acquired*). Once the infection gets a place to enlarge, it can get large enough and aggressive enough to permanently damage the heart valve in question. Yes, it can destroy valve tissue! It can also kill you!

Dr. Robert L. Shuman, a noted cardiologist, described it like this: "An abnormal valve gets endocarditis. A normal valve can get endocarditis. The valve itself provides a location for the bacteria even from normal wear and tear. That plus the turbulence of the blood flowing through the valve helps the endocarditis. If it is a bicuspid valve, endocarditis is more likely than with a tricuspid valve. A bicuspid valve is the result of a congenital defect. A tricuspid valve is normal."[ix]

How does *Staphylococcus aureus* do you in, you ask?

In order for it to change from a "nuisance bacteria" to a "killer bacteria," it needs to enter your body, go undetected, circulate through your bloodstream while you present symptoms, lodge in one or more vital organs, grow rapidly, be misdiagnosed and see no antibiotics or be the recipient of improper antibiotics which will do nothing to eliminate it from your body.

Some forms of *Staphylococcus aureus* are resistant to penicillin or to any and all penicillin-based antibiotics. These are referred to as ***Methicillin-resistant Staphylococcus aureus* or MRSA (pronounced mer-SUH).**

You test for which strain of *Staphylococcus aureus* is present by taking a blood sample for a blood culture and sensitivity. The testing needs to include the sensitivity test to determine if the strain is resistant to certain antibiotics. Otherwise, an ineffective antibiotic could be used and the infection would keep growing unchecked. Any good doctor knows this. The medical literature is substantial in this area.

How bad can MRSA be?

On January 18, 2007, Reuters Health and Science Editor Maggie Fox reported that one really bad staph germ circulating in and out of hospitals emits a poison that can kill pneumonia patients within seventy-two hours. This was the result of research findings gleaned at the Texas A&M Health Science Center in Houston who led the study.[x]

The MRSA bugs mentioned in the preceding paragraph generated toxins. The poison in this case was generated by the bacteria of a certain strain of MRSA.

The article went on to say that the toxin, called PVL, can itself cause pneumonia and can kill healthy tissue.

The Reuters article continued saying two British hospital patients passed away due to the necrotizing pneumonia in December 2006. It also killed some of the immune system cells which battled it. Apparently the PVL toxin can turbo-charge an already dangerous bacteria.

The head researcher on the study added that, fortunately, patients infected with the bacteria quickly develop a high fever and astute doctors can identify it. She said that she and her colleagues were trying to put the word out and to educate people.

A successful treatment antibiotic against this MRSA bug could be doxycycline or vancomycin according to Wikipedia.

On March 16, 2012, ABC News Blogs reported that in the ongoing evolution of bacteria versus antibiotics, common infectious strains could become deadly according to Dr. Margaret Chan, Director General of the World

Health Organization. Dr. Chan felt that continued antibiotic resistance could signal "the end of modern medicine as we know it."

Singling out hospitals, Chan said that hospitals have become "hotbeds of highy resistant pathogens" (like methicillin-resistant *Staphylococcus aureus*) "increasing the risk that hospitalization kills instead of cures."[xi]

According to the symptoms of infectious bacterial endocarditis can include: fever; night sweats; heart murmur; splinter hemorrhages; coughing; Janeway lesions; positive blood culture; and emboli (blood clots).[xii]

According to Dr. Mark Amico, during a 2013 office visit, chills are often observed as a symptom of bacterial endocarditis.

*****

In 2003-2004, approximately 29% (79.8 million persons) and 1.5% (4.1 million persons) of the U.S. population was colonized in the nose with *S. aureus* and MRSA respectively.[xiii]

The December 26, 2006 online edition of *The Wall Street Journal* quoting Reuters News Service reported that *Staph. aureus* infections and other powerful infections that thrive in hospitals kill 90,000 people and result in $4.5 billion in excess costs per year according to the Centers for Disease Control and Prevention.

The article went on to explain that many hospital administrators were not aware of how expensive hospital-acquired infections were to treat.

Continuing on, the article noted a study which found that hospitals lost $27,000 for each hospital patient who became infected by a preventable infection during his hospitalization.[xiv]

Chapter 6—Six Days and Nights and a Wake-up

How do you keep from going crazy in a hospital for six days and nights as you prepare for a life-saving surgery?

*****

Shelley was everything to me during this medical crisis. She was especially adept as our "caterer" for the next six days and nights.

I had no dietary restrictions. If I was on my way out, I was going to eat like a death row inmate savoring his last meal.

On the first morning after being admitted, Shelley went downstairs to the cafeteria and brought back *real food!* There would be **no** hospital meals for me!

I dined on bacon, eggs, hot cakes—*you name it.* When lunchtime rolled around, we would have a room pow-wow and then she would take off from the hospital and make a food run for the good stuff.

The staff would be envious as Shelley showed up with lunch offerings from Burger King, Del Taco, KFC, Carl's Jr., In 'N Out Burger, Subway, etc. It all tasted so good. I was not there for heart disease or clogged arteries, so anything was fair game.

At dinnertime, we ate well every night. We enjoyed food from Chili's, Marie Callender's (for dinners and desserts), Rosie's BBQ, and Mandarin Island for Chinese food, Acapulco for Mexican, and Domino's Pizza.

In essence, we were having a party in my room for six days.

I kidded one of the nurses saying that I hoped that she knew CPR in case I started choking on a baby back rib. I told her that I would be putting myself at risk for croaking from the hospital food if I ate it.

That drew a few chuckles from her.

One or two extra staff entered my room every night when we dined, perhaps hoping for a tidbit or two from us.

Truth be known, **there was nothing wrong with the food at VHMC.**

*****

Even though Shelley was hanging in there and put on a good show for me, inside she was coming apart. She was on an emotional roller coaster.

On several occasions when I was wheeled off for a test or lab work or something, she went downstairs and outside and called her Dad, the late Jules Nayfack. Shelley confided in him how scared she was, how awful everything really was, and that she didn't know if I would make it to my surgery — let alone make it through it.

*****

Shelley and I found lots to do to pass the time and get through those six days. For instance, we told one another funny stories and she brought me some things to read.

I imitated the voices of people that she and I both knew for the humor in it. I used my hands to talk to each other (as puppets), with each hand having a different voice. I made up outrageous things that the people I was imitating would never say but did in my story.

I used my Asian voice, my Hispanic voice, my Middle Eastern voice, my Calcutta voice, my Redneck voice and a couple that I had never used before. I even used a "bullhorn" voice. I mean, if your odds maker says that you may croak, you might as well laugh it up before they use "the hook" to get you off the stage of life.

At times, Shelley referred to me as "Cousin David." The basis for that is a long, funny story but space does not permit me to give you the details.

I nicknamed Shelley, "Parnelli Shelley," after the famous car-racer Rufus "Parnelli" Jones. Shelley drove like a maniac but she was in control. She was quite talented behind the wheel. Truth be known, she was a high speed pursuit on KCBS2 waiting to happen!

On more than one occasion, Shelley drag-raced her grandfather's '56 Buick Roadmaster at San Fernando Raceway. It had milled cylinder heads (which increased the compression ratio), a dual-carb manifold and dual carbs, and a hot camshaft with trick lifters. One day at the San Fernando Raceway in Pacoima, California when she was seventeen, Shelley dropped the tranny in it just after launching from the starting line.

We were sitting around and I was teasing Shelley about her driving.

In a **police radio voice**, I did an entire routine with faux police radio calls and fake radio "squelch" about "The Martenson Woman."

That would be Shelley.

The first fake cop voice said, "Unit 54 to dispatch. I've got a Silver Toyota Highlander doing 90 in 65 confirmed on radar on the 101 North off the Conejo Grade. **It has to be The Martenson Woman!** I think that Cousin David, the escaped mental patient, is with her. Over."

Fake squelch.

The dispatcher fake cop voice said, "Calling all cars. Be on the lookout for **The Martenson Woman**. She is hopped up on Diet Coke and headed down the Conejo Grade toward Ventura in her Silver Highlander. We expect that she will stop to use a restroom. Do not apprehend until she has used the facilities. Be further advised that the notorious Cousin David is with her. He is also hopped up on Diet Coke. Over."

Fake squelch.

*****

Every night, I told some fake story or made something up for our entertainment. A couple of times, one of the nurses would hear the story *du jour* and would crack up.

Shelley and I laughed hard and often during that week. We shared some good jokes with the staff, too. Anything was fair game to avoid thinking about the pending surgery and to alleviate the boredom.

*****

One thing that I love to do is to **put people on**. When I'm in that frame of mind, people can't tell if what comes out of my mouth is true or not.

Every chance I get, no matter who it is, if I have a shot, I take it. Some of my family and friends have been victimized often. The more I can put people on, the merrier I am is the way I look at it. If I think I can get away with it with a total stranger, I will. They are absolutely the best subjects to put on, especially when I'm with someone who knows me and I make up some b.s. story. If the person with me knows what's coming, they don't give it away.

One of my favorite put-on stories goes something like this:

I was on my back on a gurney at the Surgical Center in Encino waiting for a colonoscopy. That's right, **The Big Stinkfinger**.

It seemed that everybody in the entire facility had asked me why I was there, except for the janitor. I was sick of it.

A Hispanic physician and a Caucasian RN entered the area I was in. The doctor looked at the clipboard in his hand and said, "So, Meeeester Folck—why are you here?"

I countered with "I'm here for a brain transplant. Did the donor gorilla show up yet?"

"No. There has been a change in plans," the doctor replied with a slight smile. "We're going to use a Chihuahua instead."

So I go through the procedure and make it back to the recovery room. Doc Stinkfinger, AKA, Dr. Rahbar, from somewhere in the Middle East, appears. He is wearing a sports coat that looks like crushed velvet from a woman's evening dress. Either that or it was a cheap sofa fabric from Living Spaces furniture.

In machine-gun fashion, with his Middle-Eastern accent, he told me, "We found four polyps that I biopsied before I removed them. You were not completely clean from the bowel prep. Your colon is so large that for the next one I will give you a double prescription for the prep medicine. I will see you in six months for a follow-up. Good-bye."

Gabbedy, gabbedy! Or if you prefer, "Yakety yak!"

So I get released and my daughter, Melinda, drives me to my truck, where she lets me out. I get in and start the engine.

I'm starving, so I drive to VIP's Coffee Shop in Tarzana. That's the place where Coach John Wooden liked to go to for breakfast. I used to wave to him and exchange greetings frequently.

I sit at a booth. Misty, one of the waitresses, takes my order for an omelet.

A woman who tells the world she is from Argentina is sitting in the booth next to mine and she is looking right at me. On the back of my left hand, she sees a gauze pad with tape over it where my IV from the procedure had been.

She points to it and says, "Watt hoppin?"

"I just had a brain transplant from a Chihuahua."

Totally surprised, she says, "Jew deed?!"

Misty, the waitress, who is within earshot, covers her mouth with her hand and hurries off into the kitchen, where she bursts out laughing.

Argentina Woman reflects on what I said and comes back with "Jew no, doze doctorz, day can do any ting."

*****

In spite of everything you have read so far, you won't believe what *really* happened on Saturday April 17, 2004, which was *two days* before my scheduled surgery. I don't have much memory of what happened, as you'll see. Several people helped me to piece together the events that transpired.

*****

The 17th was an uneventful day for me and everyone providing care for me. That is until Shelley came into my room at 6:30 pm. Then **all hell broke loose**.

Prior to that, with my breathing improving and my cough almost non-existent, I was on the uptick, but only to a point. After Shelley entered my room, it went downhill quickly.

*****

Have you ever seen the famous Abbott and Costello routine, "Who's on First?"

If you haven't, it's a seemingly crazy exchange between the two comedians about what is happening in a baseball game. While it makes total sense, Bud Abbott appears totally confused and Costello thinks Abbott just doesn't get it. The beginning of this story is similar.

Have you ever been with someone who showed symptoms of a stroke?

Can you tell if someone is putting you on or not?

Smiling, Shelley walked into my room and I said, "Oh, there you are. Where have you been?"

Shelley responded as if I had asked a stupid question. She had this incredulous look on her face.

"I went home to check on Sean."

I shot back with my best comeback ever, my most snappy retort. "Well, uh, where am I?"

Shelley had that look on her face that she gets when I am messing with her.

"You're in the hospital."

"Huh? What...? What hospital?"

With a little edge to her voice, she shot back, "You're in Valleydale Hospital! The one with the tall buildings on Corsoe Boulevard?"

After a hibernating pause, I inquired, "How long have I been here...?"

In a no-nonsense manner, she replied "You've been here for six days."

"Really...? Why am I here?"

Shelley, sensing that I was teasing, said "You have a *staph.* infection in your bloodstream, **DAY-VID!**"

*****

It was a running joke that whenever I said **DAY-VID** as I spoke about myself to others, I was acting like my mom getting after me as a kid. Shelley was teasing me since she thought I was teasing her.

My mom had called me **DAY-VID** whenever I was about to get in trouble or if I was being called on the carpet. If she called me DAY-VID LEW-IS, it was going to be bad. If she called me DAY-VID LEW-IS FOLCK, I was facing a lethal injection at the big house.

*****

"You need surgery to replace your aortic heart valve. The infection ate up your heart valve. Remember?!"

My jaw dropped open. I got bug-eyed. Then I got the most thunderstruck look on my face.

"Does my, does my brother know about this? Did anyone tell my kids?"

Shelley took a thoughtful step back. Then she turned and burned rubber like a 60s top-fuel dragster as she galloped toward the nurses' station.

She got the attention of a nurse and told her, "Something is terribly wrong with my boyfriend. **I think he's had a stroke!**"

That got *everyone's* attention.

Shelley said, "When I left him two hours ago, he was fine. I mean he gets crazy when he wants to be funny. But he knew everything that was going on about what happened, why he was here, and now he doesn't remember any of it!"

One of the nurses hurried into my room with Shelley. The nurse asked me questions, the kind of questions you might ask someone if you are trying to determine whether or not they have had a stroke.

The nurse was not satisfied with my responses. She called for a doctor.

The female doctor came in and asked me, "What is your name?"

"David Lewis Folck."

Pointing toward Shelley, the doctor asked, "Who is she?"

"Shelley, Shelley, Martenson. She's my girlfriend."

"When were you born?"

"In the morning."

"What is your date of birth?"

"February 4th in 1949."

"Where were you born?"

"In Ottawa General Hospital."

"What city?"

I got a quizzical look on my face.

"Where the hospital was?"

"Yes."

"Ottawa."

"Canada?"

"Kansas."

*****

Shelley recounted that all my answers were much labored. It's a good thing that she recalled the details of the incident; otherwise these pages would be blank.

87

It was a total Looney Tune conversation!

*****

The doctor asked me to count backward from one hundred by threes.

"One hundred, ninety seven..."

I strained my brain as much as I could strain it.

"Uh, ninety. Damn."

With that, I shook my head and rested my chin on my chest.

Feeling defeated, I said, "Damn it, I can't — I don't know."

*****

Shelley took the doctor outside of my room and told her that I was an absolute wiz with numbers.

She exclaimed, "Something is really wrong with his brain!"

She got misty-eyed. "Oh, God... Dave's had a stroke," she lamented.

Then Shelley started crying.

The doctor left the room, returned to the nurses' station and considered her options before deciding that I needed a "stat" CAT scan of my brain. She wanted to know what was amiss with my grey matter.

*****

I had joked on and off for years, as many of us have, that I was brain-damaged from: having kids, working at my job, being my Mom's son, growing up with my brother, sniffing glue for years (not true), and from breathing the Los Angeles smog.

Now it was about to be demonstrated to all who knew me that I was truly brain-damaged. At last, definitive evidence! I'd be in a scientific journal. Only, I wasn't thinking about that.

*****

Shelley was breaking the news to me, all over again from the opening blow *ad nauseum*. Yet, no way did she want to be the messenger about all of this.

I had been devastated by the news as it unfolded just days earlier. At that moment I was feeling bashed all over again. Occasionally I would ask, "Who?"

In other moments of brief, normal brain functioning, I would say, "They did what?" Or "Are you sure?"

The clinker was when I asked, "Do any doctors know?"

As far as a "stat" CAT scan was concerned, forget it. It was a Saturday night. Not a chance of that happening.

It would be four hours before I got that CAT scan. The reason? Well, they had to call a technician in who lived thirty-five miles from the hospital to perform the procedure.

*****

We finished eating take-out from the Mandarin Island restaurant, and then Shelley used the rest of the four hours to fill me in some more about what had transpired. She didn't leave out anything.

Finally, they wheeled me out of my room for a CAT scan of my brain. When we got upstairs, Shelley told the female technician what happened and why the doctor ordered the scan in a summary version. She also mentioned that I seemed a little better than when she first noticed that I had gone "crackers" at about 6:30 pm.

The tech said to me, "We're going to do a CAT scan of your brain. It's going to get noisy. Do you want ear plugs?"

I nodded and took the earplugs.

She kept talking. "There is a microphone inside the machine. If you need to ask me anything, or if anything is bothering you, you can let me know, ok?"

I responded with "Ok, now what part of my body are you going to look at...?"

The tech talked to Shelley out of earshot. "I can see why he is here. He is obviously confused and disoriented."

Shelley went bonkers and lost it! What was going on with me completely fractured her coconut! She was ready for a straightjacket but I was the one who needed it!

*****

Shelley told me several years later that she thought at that moment, "Oh, my God, I am going to have to spend another four hours explaining to him what happened. I'll have to say everything all over again!"

I chuckled at that comment and, at times, also laughed pretty hard while she recounted this whole story in 2007. She said that it was all serious business to her at the time it was unfolding. Now the entire situation seems so comical. We laughed as she verbally regurgitated the details. What really broke me up was when she recounted me asking the CAT scan person why I was there after the woman had just told me.

*****

A review of my CAT scan showed that, medically, there was no evidence of a stroke.

I was told that Dr. Schwinger and Dr. Soltero were called late on that Saturday night. Both were relieved at the news that there was no evidence of a stroke.

Finally, I "recovered" enough to realize that I was back and coherent.

About that time, Dr. Amico, who had also been called with the results, entered my room with a group of residents or interns from UCLA. It was midnight on Saturday.

Previous to that meeting, I had been aware that due to the delicate and fragile structure of the *Staphylococcus aureus* growth, if it broke off and caused a significant blockage to my blood flow, I could experience a stroke, heart attack, or a pulmonary embolism. All of those scenarios could be deadly.

I asked Dr. Amico, "Can I go have the surgery now?"

He said, "David, we can't do that. We can't go in until the 19th if all goes well."

"I may not make it until then, Dr. Amico."

Shelley closed her eyes and shook her head back and forth.

"We can't intubate you for your anesthetic until your lungs are clear of the pneumonia. Right now, that is not the case," he said.

"Damn it."

"David, would you mind if each of the students listened to your heart murmur? It is not a very common murmur and I would like them to hear it."

"Sure, why not," I said.

So, one by one, about a dozen wannabe doctors listened to my heart murmur. After each had finished, I got a "thank you."

Finally, they left.

*****

Now the question I asked myself was whether or not I would make it through the rest of the night.

But what had occurred?

This is where the "black art" of medicine comes in.

With all that is known about the human body from years of clinical study, sometimes it is still a "best guess" that prevails in explaining "what happens." The best guess among my medical gurus about what happened was divided into two camps of thought.

The first guess was that some of the infection that had clustered on my heart valve broke away and entered my bloodstream. The doctors referred to them as very "**minute particles**." Part of the bloodstream debris may have lodged in my brain, causing my problem with recall and memory.

The second guess was that some "fatty" tissue in my bloodstream lodged in one or more areas in my grey matter and caused the memory/recall problem that I demonstrated. Again, these were minute particles of fat.

After the "brain-damage" crisis passed, Shelley referred to me as "Fat Head."

While I was sleeping at about 1:30 am, a doctor came to my room and told Shelley that I might have a fat tumor in my brain. He said that some fatty tissue could have lodged in one part of my brain causing all the trouble.

Don't take offense to her name-calling. I took it for the humorous aspect of the words and laughed pretty hard several times. From the moment we met, Shelley and I had been able to kid each other, and this was no exception.

None of the medical people could say, definitively, what had happened. Either there was a temporary full or partial blockage of the blood flow to certain areas of my brain.

Several years later, I further reflected on the events of that night. I was left with the feeling that maybe the entire episode was a mental tapestry woven with my imagination to protect me from the reality of my situation. That is, the infection and what it did to me.

At other points in my life, I believe that my imagination implanted ideas or thoughts in my consciousness as "protective devices" to shield me from an awful truth or to help me get past some really ugly situations in my life. It happened too many times over the years to be a coincidence.

I also wondered if the memory/recall problem was in part or in whole caused by an interaction of the medications I was taking at that time. Some of the ethical prescription medications I took had some noteworthy side effects. Who knows if all of the potential interactions between them had even been discovered?

One last point is necessary. Because of the blood level of Levaquin in my body, the size of the infection decreased and hence the amount of the "debris" that could enter my bloodstream was increased.

My best guess is that particulate infectious matter got into one or more areas of my brain, causing the fake stroke stuff. I refuse to believe that I was a "fathead."

Shelley finally left but she was shot from the events of that evening. I mean she was whipped.

*****

Sunday April 18, 2004 turned out to be a better day.

That evening, I got two pieces of good news. First, my triple pneumonia was gone. Second, my white blood count was dropping. It was almost in a normal range.

That meant that the surgery was on for the morning of the next day. The doctors did not want to wait any longer.

I slept better that night buoyed by the thought of the surgery. Instead of dreading it, I looked forward to it. At last, the surgery would be done!

*****

Many times during that week prior to the surgery, I felt that it wasn't really me asking medical questions, and wanting to read the medical reports and lab results. If it was not me, then who was it?

I've come to think it was the deceased Marilyn Folck re-entering my world and making the inquiries. Her spirit was watching over me.

Chapter 7—Screw the Grim Reaper

Hospital personnel were everywhere in my room after I woke up on Monday April 19th. I felt better than I had when I was admitted on the 12th. However, I was still very ill.

In my mind, Dr. Amico, Dr. Schwinger and Dr. Soltero were "The Three Wise Men" in my drama.

My mindset about what lead up to this day was this: If I'm going down, I'm taking as many of my enemies with me as I can. It was my combat veteran's mentality coming into play.

My blood infection had cleared substantially and my lungs were clear. The "fix" on my care was in. No one was going to lose me on their "watch."

If anything, I was more concerned about *not* having the surgery. The "faux" stroke had not set too well with me.

I was not scared.

When I decide on something, it is an all-in bet. I don't waver. I go for it.

I looked down. The trunk of my body was as hairless as a newborn's. I had quite a bit of mileage and my "sheet metal" was stretched a bit more than it had been when I left the factory. I had dings all over. A little Bondo and some touch-up paint wouldn't take care of those things.

The anesthesiologist gave me my anesthetic in my room before I got into the operating room. I went out very quickly.

*****

Some months after the surgery, I reviewed all the medical bills and saw how many people were getting paid to assist in my surgery. I would later learn that the OR had a plethora of monitoring devices when my surgery began. My guess was that it looked like a NASA control room for one of the space shuttle missions.

*****

The surgery took several hours to complete as it was complex.

I had been in full bypass for about two hours in surgery. In my mind, it meant that I was alive but not living.

My blood had been cooled down with an icy saline solution while I was on bypass. My body temperature was also kept low during the surgery.

Dr. Soltero actually debrided the vegetation on my heart valve by hand with special surgical tools. He did the aortic valve change out after some patching in the aortic root.

At that point I got a jumpstart, achieved a normal heart rhythm, had no problems with leakage and was closed up using three woven strands of copper wire for thread. Finally, I was living again.

By the way, there were **two kinds of bacteria infecting my body upon further review of lab cultures** taken during the surgery. The Levaquin killed the virulent strain of *Staphylococcus aureus* in my blood but did not eradicate the second aggressive, very rare bacterium which was also methicillin-resistant. Dr. Soltero did that with the debridement.

There will be more on this strain later.

*****

Post-surgery, the scene was rather solemn for my family and girlfriend as I started to come to in the recovery room. My eyelids flickered. Then they flickered some more.

Shelley exclaimed, "He opened his eyes. Dave, can you hear me?"

I moved my right hand slightly.

"Good," she said softly. Shelley grabbed my hand and chimed in with "My God, you made it!"

She summoned my brother, Forrest, to come in.

Forrest recounted that I looked like **the aftermath of a mad scientist's experiment** that had gone wrong. You know, like you might see in an old black and white sci-fi/horror film.

I was intubated, and tape covered one of my eyes, which gave me a Cyclops-like appearance. Intravenous lines were in both arms. I couldn't talk.

My brother told me months later that I also looked like a "Gomer" at that moment. You know. That's the look a patient gets just before he flat lines and his heart monitor sounds a steady "beeeeeeeeeeeeeeeep!"

Then someone shouts, "Paddles! Give me 500 watts. Clear!" And the patient bucks like a bronco from the electric current that zaps through him from head to toe.

Yet I wasn't dreaming. I **had survived** open-heart surgery. Living or dying was no longer an issue for me.

The Grim Reaper had gotten his ass kicked!

I didn't move too much at first. Then I felt a natural urge.

"Ummmmmmmmmmm," I said.

Shelley asked, "What was that?"

"Ummmmmmmmmmmmmmmmmmmmmmmmm!"

My brother said, "It's Dave."

My uncovered eye was bulging as I tried to communicate.

Shelley asked, "What does he want?"

"UMMMMMMMMMMMMMMMMMMMMMMMMMMMM!"

Being the guy that he is, Forrest offered up, "I think he needs to pee."

"UMMMMMMMMMMMMMMM.
UMMMMMMMMMMMMMMMMM. UMMMMMMMMMMMM!"

"Yeah, that's it; that's what he wants," my brother said.

After being summoned to my bedside, one of the recovery room nurses told me, "Go. You're wearing a catheter."

I let her rip! It felt so good and it was a long pee. Finally my bladder was empty.

A little later, a doctor removed the tube from my throat and mouth and the tape covering my eye. No more Cyclops in the room.

*****

Two transportation techs wheeled me to the cardiac ICU once I was fully awake. In my new bed, I remember looking myself over and seeing tubes everywhere and leads for various monitoring devices. Electronic monitors decorated the room.

Still, I could tell that **everything was fine with my heart**. I hadn't been told anything, but I could tell. I had gone toe to toe with The Grim Reaper and had beaten him into submission.

*****

I think it was my daughter Melinda who called her half-sister — my third child, Jessica — after the surgery.

My relationship with Jessica had gotten a bit strained when she left my home to live with her mom, my second "ex", outside of Dallas. It wasn't the fact that Jessica wanted to live with her mom; it was how she went about it and the timing of it that had irritated me.

While my brother and Shelley were in my room, the phone on my nightstand rang. I was engaged in a conversation with one of the hospital staff, so Forrest answered the phone.

He said, "Hello. Jessie! How are you? Your dad is here. He's doing great. The surgery went well."

The two of them chatted for a few minutes. Then my brother put his hand over the mouthpiece to the phone.

"Dave? Jessie wants to talk to you."

We did the Father-Daughter chit-chat thingy for a few minutes. Jessie volunteered that she was really scared about the idea of my open-heart surgery.

I told her that I was in pain but otherwise ok.

"Dad, there is someone here who wants to talk to you" Jessie said.

"Hello?" I said.

Oh, my God!! It was my second ex, Connie, an RN. We had not parted on good terms; however, I had seen her, post-divorce, at a couple of family affairs for Jenasis and Elijah, my Granddaughter and Grandson.

As was sometimes her custom whenever she dissolved a relationship with another person, Connie trashed me when we divorced. At least she tried to do that. On that day in the ICU, I just let her go on and on.

I made small talk with her, **very small talk**. Then Connie asked me, "Do you need Jessie and me to come out and help you?"

I couldn't believe what she had just asked me!

Always wanting to be in the spotlight, Connie was looking for her opportunity. She was always the same.

Perhaps her professional callings had reared up. My guess was that she also wanted to do something for me. Over many years toward the end of our marriage, I had cared for her when her autoimmune disorder was so out of control.

Connie was a very good nurse during her working years. During her career, she helped a lot of people in the labor and delivery units where she had worked and also as a perinatology nurse. My ex was very good at what she did.

But I was not pregnant, and I was not in labor.

"No, you don't need to come out," I uttered.

I was as diplomatic as humanly possible under the circumstances.

I could feel my heart rate increasing and it showed on the monitor.

My palms began to sweat at the thought of her being physically near me again. My blood pressure was rising as well. I simply could not have her here with me!

I wanted nothing to do with Connie post-divorce and I still don't.

I said good-bye and handed the phone back to my brother, whispering emphatically to him, "**Tell her NOT to come out!**"

Then I made all kinds of gestures to indicate "No." I shook my head back and forth, I ran my right index finger across my throat, and I made an "X" with my arms. I said the word, "Nyet!"

Shelley laughed out loud. "You're too funny," she said.

My brother smiled as he looked at me with my bug eyes. He put his hand to his heart and feigned heart trouble. I wanted to smack him! Son of a bitch.

He talked with Connie like the Dutch uncle he can be when needed and told her three times not to come out. Then he handed me the phone saying, "Its Jessie."

Before I spoke to Jessica one more time, I reflected that I had just dodged a bullet by keeping my ex in Texas.

I talked with my daughter for a few more moments. Jessie was shaken but she had her mother with her for support. She said that her grandmother, Ruth Eickel, sent her best to me.

I told Jessie to thank Ruth, who I adored. She had been a wonderful Mother-in-Law for about sixteen years.

I also mentioned to Jessica that she was welcome to come to California to see me if she came alone. She chuckled a little and didn't say anything in response to that. I told her that I would call with details when I had them to give. Then I told Jessie that I did not know how long I would be in the coronary care ICU. She seemed satisfied. Finally, I finished the phone call.

Shortly after that, my heart rate went back to a safe range and my blood pressure went down to a normal range as well. I rolled my eyes. If the surgery hadn't killed me, a phone call from my second ex might have!

I looked at my brother and Shelley and said, "Don't say a thing!"

Both of them were smiling. My daughter Melinda chuckled.

It was then that I imagined a front page story in the *Los Angeles Daily News* that said something like this: "Yesterday, a post-surgical heart patient died of a massive cardiac arrest after his ex-wife called offering to take care of him."

*****

Dr. Soltero entered my room still in his scrubs. He said, "The surgery went well. You got the human tissue valve, which is what we had hoped for. Your aortic root was infected and slightly damaged by the infection. No need to be concerned about it. I repaired it and it looked good after the repair."

I nodded my head up and down slightly.

"Your heart was in very good shape from what I saw once it was open. No sign of any heart disease, nothing. Whatever you've been doing over the years for exercise and diet has worked very well. I saw the whole inside of your heart. The infection did not enter any of your heart chambers."

101

As I recalled this, I reflected about a life of vigorous exercise. All those years in my twenties and thirties when I had been an avid jogger came back to me. After that, I recalled years of bike riding about five days a week. All of that had paid off.

Soltero continued and said, "From all the lab readings and monitor indications, I can tell you now that you have a normally functioning heart in every way. Nothing is amiss with your heart right now. We waited for a while to make sure that there was no post-surgical bleeding of any kind before we closed. We're going to keep an eye on you for a few days."

After that, Dr. Soltero left my room.

*****

Shelley came in and walked up to me. She squeezed my hand and I squeezed back.

She said, "Your brother was really shook up after he saw you in the recovery room. He went out of the room into the corridor and cried. I think he cried for five minutes or so. It really got to him."

My brother and I were the only ones left from our family of four: Jean, Marilyn, Forrest, David. My Mom and Dad had both left this world. The thought of me kicking off had been heavily on Forrest's mind since I told him that I had been hospitalized. He had driven up from San Diego to be with me when my chest was cut open. He stayed a little while longer and then he left the hospital.

Melinda came back in. She became tearful as we spoke. I could tell that it was all too much for my daughter seeing me like I was. She didn't stay long.

"Dad, I'm glad that you made it. I think that you made all the right choices since you got here. Don't leave me. I still need you in my life."

We hugged and then she left. She couldn't take it. Having me check out at age fifty-five was not in her plans.

Dr. Schwinger came by. He said, "Congratulations. Your new valve is working great. I'm very pleased with the outcome for your sake. We need to monitor your urine output and a few other things for a few days, ok?"

We chatted a little more and he left.

My spirits and mood were both elevated. Overall, I felt like about a 4 on a scale of 1 to 10.

Dr. Amico made an appearance.

I asked, half-mocking him, "You aren't going to listen to my heart murmur, are you?"

"No. No need for that. Problem solved! You look so much better. I'll stop in every day while you're here."

*****

Then "**The Turk**" came in.

"The Turk" was my nickname for ANY respiratory therapist (RT).

Oh, say your prayers if you ever have to deal with "The Turk" post-surgery! He might kill you immediately following your surgery and your obituary might say, in part, "He/she died in a hospital bed due to a respiratory arrest while using a post-surgical breathing device."

On that visit, the tech had a breathing device which he showed me and talked about. I was less than enthusiastic about the idea of using it.

It was not the device that got to me; it was what I had to do with it that almost did me in.

I thought to myself, "Can we get a stunt double for me? I can pay good money!"

I didn't know it then, but for the next month I would be driven somewhat crazy trying to regain my full lung capacity. The pneumonia had left

103

my lungs at less than full capacity. That was one of the reasons for using the breathing device.

Another reason was to prevent the onset of a post-surgical lung infection from fluid pooling in my lungs.

Blow, blow, blow, blow and blow some more. Using that damn device wore me out.

The first time I blew into that tube, I damn near croaked. I was very disappointed that I had barely moved the little ball inside the device with my exhalations.

I tried to put the discomfort from using the device out of my mind. I survived the surgery, but would "The Turk" have the last laugh?

I conjured up absolutely evil thoughts about the RT. I wanted him to wear that breathing device on a part of his lower anatomy where the moon didn't shine!

When he finally left, I pulled the covers all the way up and over my head.

If I resembled a corpse on a table in a room full of coroner's cadavers, that's what I intended. I wanted to die.

I imagined "The Turk" to be some Nazi from a 1940s war movie. You know, where some war prisoner is being interrogated by an SS officer played by Peter Lorre wearing a monocle. During the interrogation, the prisoner sits on a simple wooden chair beneath a bare light bulb hanging down from the ceiling.

The Nazi in the film would say something like "You half relatiffs in (*fill in the blank*)? Vee half vays to deel wit chew!"

Then the Nazi would blow cigarette smoke into the prisoner's face, causing a "Hack, hack, hack" from the prisoner.

I'm positive that "The Turk" wanted to say to me, "You have breathing problems at Valleydale Hospital? We have ways to deal with that." But he didn't. Even so, the breathing tube would be shoved in my face, and I would make an attempt to eject a lung or two for a new world distance record every time I used it.

*****

Shelley managed to stay that first night in the room. The staff ignored the fact that she was not a family member.

Early on the morning of the 20th, I had a nightmare. It was a 10 on a scale of 1 to 10, 10 being the worst.

The Grim Reaper came after me in a haunting, frightening scene courtesy of my vivid imagination. The hooded killer kept coming closer to me as I saw myself lying on a crude operating table from the Dark Ages all alone in a candlelit cave. Finally, I flailed my arms and legs and screamed at the figure yelling, "Screw you!"

I woke up after pushing and kicking my bed table onto its side. My fresh incision hurt like hell!

An aide who heard the commotion while at the nurses station came in and meekly asked, "Are you ok?"

With my folded arms hugging my chest, I groaned from the pain.

"No" was all I said.

She rushed out of the room.

Shelley came to my side to comfort me.

After the surgical procedure, I was given narcotic-based pain killers. When you have your breastbone cut open with a cutting wheel, and then they stitch you up with three-strand braided copper wires, you need very strong medication to dull the pain. Demerol and Morphine had been flowing into me.

I remember getting Demerol just before I went to sleep on the evening of the 19th. I was already depressed from the underlying PTSD.

105

Opiate analgesics, like Demerol, depress your central nervous system to hide the physical pain you are feeling from your conscious thoughts. It's a con game for your mind courtesy of the narcotics.

Turns out that the Demerol heightened my depression and the result was a nightmare. For someone besieged by a sleep disorder, this was the last straw. The battle lines were drawn.

Shelley was asked to leave by the hospital staff. She left my room at about 9:00 am and went home.

*****

Shortly after Shelley left, a pain control specialist came into my room. She was the person responsble for all pain meds that were dispensed on the unit. Trust me when I say I gave it her!

With an edgy voice, I yelled at her saying, "I don't want that crap anymore. It made me crazy beyond belief last night. I don't want **any more** of it!"

"You still have significant pain at this point and the doctor..." she said.

Cutting her off in mid-sentence, I said "Get me some high-performance aspirin. Anything but that! I'm crazy to begin with and that stuff makes me crazier!"

The head nurse dashed into the room near the end of the conversation. She told me, "It is best that you take the Demerol."

So I simply repeated my tirade about narcotic analgesics to her. I said, "I can tolerate ANY pain but not the side effects of the Demerol! If you are too dense to understand that, then get someone else in here to take care of me. Put it on my chart that I am refusing any more Demerol. Got it?!"

They hurried out of my room and then I cried. For the first time since I had been admitted to the hospital, I cried. It lasted a good ten minutes. My chest throbbed as I cried.

I did not take any more narcotic analgesics for the remainder of my stay at VHMC. As a result, I didn't have any other nightmares during my stay. My intuition had been correct about the Demerol.

*****

A little later on April 20th, things were not looking too good for me on several fronts. First, my weight was up twelve pounds compared to my pre-surgical weight.

Also, my Three Wise Men had grown concerned about the lack of renal output. My kidneys seemed be on a break.

They ended their summit in my room. About ten minutes later, an RN came in and gave me Lasix, a potent diuretic. I learned that it was quite common in post-heart-surgery cases for Lasix to be given to the patient to jump start his/her renal discharge system.

About forty-five minutes after taking the pill, I peed like Man O'War. It was like Niagara Falls in my room. I cut loose. I pissed up a storm. I should have moved my bed into the bathroom. For the next two days, if the staff wanted me, they could have found me in the can!

I have remained on a daily dose of Lasix for years as, post-surgically, I had congestive heart failure. Without the Lasix, I puffed up from excess fluid retention.

I lost the new twelve pounds in two days after I started taking Lasix.

*****

What is there to do in a coronary ICU?

You greet the stampede of medical personnel coming into your room.

As soon as you are able, you offer them money to get you out of the hospital by taking you out the back way. You say to them that you are willing to shinny down tied-together bedsheets to get out of the place. You offer any amount to hide in a soiled linen cart. You offer a guy from the kitchen money to hide you in the food service cart. Etc., etc., etc.

*****

All kidding aside, I was well cared for in the coronary ICU at VHMC. Nevertheless, I was anxious to leave.

Later that day, I was transferred to a regular post-op med-surgical ward. Post-op — except for the run-in with the pain control people and the need for Lasix — everything went well.

And that is how you can feel so good before and after open-heart surgery.

Chapter 8—I Get My Walking Papers

Recovery from an open-heart surgery requires physical and emotional strength and fortitude. In my case, I had to find ways to allow myself to smile, as it was a difficult process that awaited me.

*****

When I awoke on Friday April 23, 2004, I felt like a 5 on a scale of 1 to 10, 10 being best.

Yes, I was depressed deep down from the entire experience. I tried not to focus on that, though, since the medical danger from the incident had passed. My brain was working and I was gaining strength. There would be no stroke or heart attack in my future, at least not from this crisis.

I remember sitting on the edge of the bed and wondering, "Is this really happening? Am I getting my life back?"

I looked down the front of my body after untying the hospital gown. I saw a "zipper" right down the middle of my chest. I touched the surgical scar. At that point I realized that what had happened was very real. None of it had been a dream. I ran my right index finger down the length of the scar. A moment later, tears welled up in my eyes.

I was a survivor once again in this life. I had experienced that feeling before.

I got up and shuffled through several corridors on the floor. I was doing my daily walk.

Then, as the sun began its rise in the eastern sky, I managed to see the real world outside. On the roof of the hospital tower I was in, I got some breaths of fresh air as I walked around. I sat in a chair at one of the tables on the roof that was part of a patio. I enjoyed the feeling of the morning sun on my face.

About fifteen minutes later, I made it back to my room. I disrobed and took a shower — a real shower! The warm water cascaded from the top of my head down my body.

I must have stayed under the water for fifteen or twenty minutes, which was a world record for me. My normal shower length was about five minutes. I learned to take short showers when I was in the Army.

I toweled off. I did not put my gown back on and climbed back into bed wearing only my briefs.

*****

At about 10 o'clock that morning, The Three Wise Men came into my room for a conference. Each of the doctors said that there was no reason why I needed to continue my hospital stay. All of my labs, test results, etc. said that it was time to release me.

I broke into a smile and thanked them. The only things left to do were to endure a few more blood draws, another EKG strip, two more breathing treatments, and vital signs times 3.

I also had a PICC (peripherally inserted central catheter) line installed in the hospital Radiology Department. A doctor (can't recall his name) installed the line by entering a vein in my left arm and sliding the catheter all the way into my heart. Neat trick and it cost a pretty penny.

Once the device was installed, daily doses of antibiotics and other drugs I would need for the next month could be injected at the end of the PICC line in my arm. The antibiotic and drug regimens were mandatory post heart valve surgery. The antibiotics would go directly into my heart.

The doctor finished his work and left. A nurse came in and gave me a quick class about how I could perform maintenance on the line. "No way," I thought.

I said to her, "That won't work with me."

110

I was not thinking clearly for one thing and there were a lot of steps involved. For another thing, the maintenance was to lessen the likelihood of an infection.

A damn infection had almost killed me, and I did not want to take the responsibility for taking care of the line and catching another infection. I stood my ground.

When I got back to my room, I asked Dr. Schwinger to write an order for a home healthcare nurse to come to my house to keep the PICC line working. I conveyed to him how difficult it would be for me to take care of the line since I was depressed and because my fine motor skills were not that good, not at age fifty-five.

He concurred and wrote the order.

*****

Finally, in the early afternoon, my parole papers arrived. I was already dressed to make a quick exit. I called Shelley, and she told me that she would get there around 5:00 pm since she had gone in to work. She needed to do some filings in the federal court in downtown Los Angeles.

In his report titled "DISCHARGE," Dr. Shalita noted:

"FINAL DIAGNOSIS:

1. PNEUMONIA; TREATED AND RESOLVED.
2. STAPHYLOCOCCUS AUREUS ENDOCARIDITIS; BEING TREATED AND STABLE.
3. SEPTICEMIA SECONDARY TO THE ABOVE; TREATED AND RESOLVED.
4. AORTIC INSUFFICIENY/REGURGITATION; SURGICAL CORRECTION VIA AVR, STABLE.
5. CONGESTIVE HEART FAILURE; TREATED AND STABLE.
6. POST-TRAUMATIC STRESS DISORDER; CHRONIC IN STABLE CONDITION.

*****

Shelley arrived at the hospital on time. Yes, there is a first for everything in this world.

We drove to Rosie's BBQ in Northridge for dinner. The smells there were heavenly. Yes, food with high fat content, real French fries with salt, and some diet sodas laced with caffeine would be just the ticket, even if my heart skipped a beat.

We drove back to my place in Reseda. As soon as Shelley's car got within fifty feet of my front parking strip, my four cats (Max, Sugar, Thelma and Louise) loped from the front of the house to the parking strip, having seen me in her car.

Shelley parked and turned off the engine. Max, my 17+ pound long-haired tuxedo cat, hopped into the cab of the Highlander and then right onto my lap when I opened the door to get out. He jammed his head into my stomach. I spent several minutes petting him.

The other cats were serenading me from the parking strip. I face butted Max a couple of times before I finally got out of the car.

Shelley cracked up.

I shuffled to the front porch. Each of my cats rubbed my legs.

*****

Whenever my brother Forrest feels like the crap is hitting the fan in his life, he reacts by cleaning something. Anything and everything are fair game:

cars, houses, driveways, the dishes, and even laundry. He cleans, cleans and cleans.

The running joke between us was that when he had marital problems with his first wife, their house had never looked so clean. He took it out on the house. There was no dust anywhere, and every waste basket was emptied every day and the house was free of debris.

As soon as I walked in, I could tell that Forrest had been there and had done his thing. Every room in my place was clean, neat and tidy. I was grateful to say the least. I certainly didn't have the energy to do it myself.

*****

After Shelley left, I was alone with my thoughts. I never did turn the lights on, and I stayed in the living room way past the time that the sun goes down alone with my thoughts.

I bawled my eyes out in a major cry fest. After about a half an hour of that, I pulled myself together.

I knew that what had happened to me over the past twenty-seven days was painfully true, both physically and emotionally. I was a wreck in all ways. Some part of me was still in shock and disbelief.

I tried not to go too deeply into that black hole of negative thoughts because, collectively, those thoughts were overwhelming. Instead, I prompted my consciousness to invite good thoughts about the episode into my head.

The Three Wise Men and the supporting staff at VHMC had been magnificent. I had made the right choice to stay at VHMC and not go to UCLA.

I pushed all of the right buttons, yanked on the right levers and pulled the cords that led to a medical success.

Still, I sat in my darkened living room for hours before I went to bed.

That night, 5 O'clock Charlie laid low. I guessed that he was tired, too.

*****

Shortly after I got up on Saturday, I went to my computer to check my emails. I had a ton of them in my inbox.

I wrote some to co-workers at my office in Calabasas, California. Within a few minutes of writing them, my phone was ringing off the hook.

I fielded three calls from work friends who were all shocked but pleased that I had survived. I even got a call from my former boss, Nancy. She was at a loss for words. I comforted her that I would be ok, that it would take some time to heal and thanked her, again, for giving me the heads-up on the changes at our office in January. That was what prompted me to go on disability back then.

One of my claims rep pals said that obviously someone had really screwed up. He advised me to get an attorney and look into the whole situation. He said, "I don't think you can let this go."

*****

After a couple of hours, I had had enough of that. I got up and got my shoes on. I dragged my intravenous pole outside with me, the one that held bags of IV meds and allowed for my antibiotics to treat me, and headed for the sidewalk.

My four cats joined me and clowned around the whole time.

Feeling full of energy, I headed North on Aura Avenue. I was moving at a snail's pace, but I was moving.

I made it six houses to the north of my place before I stopped to rest.

For the next few days, every time I walked, the cats came along. It was like a party each time. They chased each other, chased bugs and flying insects, rolled in patches of dirt, and jumped over small hedges all of which caused me to smile and chuckle. Their antics were welcome because the reality of recovering from open-heart surgery was pretty awful.

I told Shelley about it, and she came on the second morning and witnessed their clowning. She couldn't believe it. She thought that I had made it up.

*****

After I got back from my walk on Sunday April 25th, Shelley and I went to the ER at Valleydale because I was not doing well.

On the Emergency Department Sign-in Sheet, I wrote, "Post-op open heart surgery 4/19/04. Shortness of breath, fluid build-up in lungs." That was at 9:48 am.

The problem was that I did not have a prescription for Lasix or a Lasix equivalent. Ann McKittrick, MD was the attending physician and she gave me a prescription for Lasix, which I had filled.

I got back home. About an hour after I took it, I urinated like there was no tomorrow. I continued to pee, on and off, for several hours.

My condition improved.

*****

I saw Dr. Amico the following Monday. He had lab results, as I had gotten a blood draw just before leaving the hospital.

I was instructed to take Lasix, eat oranges or bananas, and refer to a sheet I was given for other foods with potassium in them as my level was low.

I took it easy for the rest of the day. Reality had reared its head again. My recovery would not be a straight line thing.

*****

And what about my knee?

Spending all that time off my feet helped my knee. The swelling had gone away, but some discomfort was noticeable. Since I wasn't walking far at this point, my knee was not aggravated very much.

When you recover from a serious medical problem, you have to weave in everything else that is going on in your world. You have to find time for everything. The ordinary day-to-day parts of your life don't go away.

I had not had a regular exercise regimen since December 27, 2003. I was out of shape. That only made the physical recovery more difficult.

*****

There was no particular rule book to go by for my recovery, save for the instructions I received from the various home healthcare nurses. They kept my PICC line clean and in good shape, changed the bandages and dressings associated with it, gave me my meds and so forth.

I remember being home that second weekend. Shelley was there when the home healthcare nurse came for her visit.

The home healthcare nurse decided to try to convince me to take care of the PICC line all by myself. I was in a terrible depression and I was not retaining information well, yet she got right into how I could flush out the line and everything by myself.

I watched her and so did Shelley. We were both overwhelmed by how involved the process was.

"I wouldn't want to try this by myself," Shelley said.

"I can't do that. It's too confusing," I told the nurse. "You totally lost me five minutes ago. I don't think you realize how depressed I am." The nurse finally threw in the towel on all of that.

*****

In spite of a respite from the knee woes, my lack of sleep was bothersome. My sleep was not restful and not long at night. I also had side effects from some of the meds I took post-op.

I especially did not like the side effects of the anti-hypertension medication that I took, Atenonol. It was prescribed to keep my blood pressure down.

Atenonol was not user-friendly for me. It caused me to have an occasional shortness of breath, and slowed down, uneven and irregular heartbeats. It heightened my depression, gave me cold hands and feet, decreased my sex drive, and produced mild tremors in my hands after exercise.

Hypertension is the main symptom any cardiologist worries about in a post open-heart surgical patient. At the first sign of high blood pressure, they run tests on you and put you on a medication for it.

While I was on that med, every time I rose from lying down or sitting, I got light-headed. It slowed my heart rate. At times, I felt dizzy from taking it. It interjected another layer of "fog" into my brain. It was just what I didn't need.

Atenonol slows down your blood flow in the hope that it will reduce the likelihood of a stroke. Dealing with the realities of that drug — all of them, collectively, made living with it a royal pain.

117

It was anything but delightful to ride a bicycle, exercise vigorously, bowl, and do household chores after taking it.

The effects of Atenonol almost broke my spirits. I never felt so restricted by any one medication in my life. It made me feel less interested in life — period.

I didn't give in to the side effects. I pushed ahead. Intellectually, I knew that the side effects were part of the price of keeping my heart in check for a while. On the other hand, I didn't miss Atenonol one iota when I finally got off of it some months later.

*****

The surgical scar was painful. And that pain lasted for quite some time.

After any surgery, your body needs at least a month for any area that was cut or rejoined to knit back together.

When you get a chest job, as I mentioned previously, there is also a need to take deep breaths for weeks afterward.

Yes, I had a new "Turk" who visited me at home every day — the home healthcare RN. I got so sick of that damn breathing tube. Whenever I used it, it put pressure on my surgical scar. It was a double whammy.

Mentally, I went through my entire library of profanity at least five times whenever I blew. Near the end of the breathing exercises, I was on the cusp of bringing some new profanity into the world.

I never took out my aches and pains on any of the people who helped me. I kept it all inside. I just went about my post-surgical tasks. It was right for me to be civil to them but I didn't really want to be that way.

*****

Conflicts raged within me about my whole state of affairs. I knew that it was all for my own good, yet I was borderline for a long time about descending into the "Black Hole of Depression" while I pushed myself. I did not want to go there because I sensed that it was a deep hole.

I did everything I could to avoid it. This wasn't easy. It's one thing if you have heart surgery from the results of poor eating habits, a congenital defect, a sedentary lifestyle or aging. It is quite another if someone causes your need for it.

I fought the depression, and I didn't want to get to the angry feelings underlying the depression. I became the "Good David," essentially turning my cheek about the angry feelings that I had. I needed my energy for other things, instead of anger.

With the post-surgical chest scar, I missed one particular activity that I had enjoyed immensely since age ten. I could not let a cat lie on my chest without a lot of pain and discomfort.

As a guy who loves cats and loves to have a cat be so physically close for the enjoyment that I get out of it, I felt that I simply couldn't tolerate this. Yet I had to give the activity up for a while.

My cats weren't happy about it either.

I was coping with a myriad of obstacles in my life as I recovered. Some days, it all seemed so overwhelming.

*****

Walking after my surgery saved me. I so looked forward to it. I could count on my legs carrying me in spite of my knee issues.

The neighbors queried me about the wheeled intravenous pole that tagged along with me. I filled them in on what had happened.

119

I could gauge my progress by how much farther I could walk each day from the previous day. It was simple; if I beat my previous world record, then I must be getting better.

On those first few mornings, I was very slow and I didn't go very far. A few houses down the block and I would be leaking oil from at least two cylinders. Hard breathing was not desirable either. And that came with the territory early on. I tried not to exert myself too much.

I eked out gains every day. Mentally, I pushed myself to achieve better, even though I didn't always want to.

I did miss walking a few days in the first two weeks I was home because I was so damn tired, tired of everything.

By the end of the second week, I could walk one square block. At the end of the third week, two square blocks. By four weeks, four square blocks.

After a month, the home healthcare nurses no longer needed to see me. The intravenous antibiotics were no longer necessary. The PICC line and PICC line maintenance were kaput. The goddamn breathing treatments were only a memory. I did require the anti-hypertension medication on a daily basis, which sucked.

There were post-surgical medical appointments to contend with, The Three Wise Men, lab techs, blood draws, EKGs, x-rays, questions, scans, Cupid, Donner and Blitzen. Everyone who wanted a piece of me inspected my skin, fingernails, and the incision. It seemed endless.

I should have negotiated a lifetime pass for the parking lot at the one medical building I went to so many times. Either that or I should have purchased a designated parking spot. All of my doctors were there. So I went to this place frequently.

Your privacy is invaded to the max before, during and after open-heart surgery. Privacy is not private anymore. You abdicate your privacy to give yourself every opportunity to make a full recovery.

Some other people had caused all of this to happen to me, not me. I wanted to kick the crap out of someone.

My toes were full of blisters from walking for six weeks. I came to the conclusion that I needed to start riding my bicycle rather than walk.

*****

I got on my bike and made the substitution. I managed a twenty-minute bike ride that first day. My calves and thighs were on fire afterward.

Pumping your legs via bike riding really gets the blood flowing. It is wonderful for your circulation.

I got to know the streets in my neighborhood quite well. I knew where every pothole was on every street as well as every house that was for sale. I knew all the cars in the neighborhood.

By late June, I was riding ten miles a day on my bike. That is roughly equivalent to a one-hour ride at a modest clip. My thigh muscles were feeling like steel cables at that point.

Then my right knee started "barking." What was healthy in one sense was a downhill slide of discomfort in another.

My knee wasn't my only bothersome symptom...

Chapter 9—Permanent Disabilities

I had been feuding with the Department of Veterans Affairs for over a year believing that I was 100% disabled from the effects of my PTSD. They kept denying me that level of disability. They rated me at 60% disabled. I thought that they were pricks.

The collective behavior of that agency, particularly those that held the rating purse strings, was disgraceful. Their own independent psychiatrist had offered up that I was 100% disabled and they ignored his findings.

Meanwhile, my near-death incident had evoked some very strong feelings deep inside me about my basic survival. Like the aftermath of a bad meal, they kept coming back.

*****

For one thing, my sleep situation was an absolute hairball. My sleep disruption had gotten worse.

I got a consult at the V.A. Medical Center in West Los Angeles for a sleep study. They put me on a waiting list. I realized that I would not have the study done for a while. This was a small facility with limited patient capacity and a long waiting list.

I did not want to take any prophylactic meds for my sleep problem until I knew specifically what it was. Because of that, 5 O'clock Charlie was my bedmate every morning.

I napped every day to make up both for my lost sleep and my interrupted sleep. The physical workout of the blowing and breathing and more blowing and breathing was tiring. By 1:30 or 2:00 pm every day, I was napping.

Most of the time, it was a very light sleep. Not that deep refreshing REM sleep, the one that lets you get up and face the world with a decent attitude.

During my initial recovery, performing activities of daily living proved difficult. These included cooking, household chores, grocery shopping, dining out, and going to a movie. All of those activities required energy. I had an energy crisis plain and simple, and my house was a mess.

I tried to maintain my personal hygiene since that was important to fighting infection. However, I was not up to my usual standards.

I had no time for hobbies and no energy for them either.

With my new extended life, I had thoughts of picking up all kinds of new activities: building a race car, woodworking, restoring an old car. All of those thoughts were pervasive. They further clouded my mind.

I tried to push those thoughts and others to the sidelines in order to cope with my new reality. The results were mixed.

*****

I went up on my antidepressants on the advice of my psychiatric resident at the Sepulveda V.A.M.C. They kept my emotions and mental state propped up.

Even with the increased meds, it still wasn't great for me as far as decision-making, and I often felt overwhelmed. Life was still coming at me pretty hard. I cried, too.

I never had any suicidal ideation or other suicidal thoughts after I got home from the hospital. Thoughts of life and living permeated my consciousness.

Earlier in my life on several occasions, I dealt with suicidal ideation. Fortunately, I never physically harmed myself on any of those occasions.

I remember one occasion when I wanted to drive my car into a freeway underpass column. I was all set to leave my house but I had a dead battery. I pulled myself together, hiked to a parts store and back with a new battery, installed it and drove to the V.A. for a consult.

123

When I could not block it post-surgery, I re-lived the build-up to the operation in my head. It was not pleasant.

Thoughts of legal recourse over my plight were becoming more and more common. I pushed them out of my mind. I made a decision that I would respond to them at a later time if that was what I wanted to do.

*****

I finally came to a decision with Dr. Friedland regarding my knee. We agreed that whenever I got medical releases from The Three Wise Men, I would have the arthroscopic surgery I so desperately needed.

After one of the visits to his office, Dr. Friedland asked me to tell him what had happened. I filled him in the best that I could, even though I had incomplete knowledge. I must have talked to him for half an hour non-stop.

He was aghast at what had happened and all the ridiculous excuses that were offered by those who were involved. He said, "It never should have happened. A first-year medical student wouldn't have done any of that!"

*****

I took an aspirin every day post-surgically. It was prescribed to decrease the probability of forming a blood clot. But I got nosebleeds from taking the aspirin. They were a nuisance but a necessary evil. I put up with them but the nosebleeds came at the most inopportune times.

Because I had a human tissue valve, I did not require a blood thinner like Coumadin. The drug Coumadin would have limited what activities I could have done.

With Coumadin, if you fell or sustained a bruise of any kind, your blood would not clot like it did normally — giving you larger bruises or hematomas. I had seen that happen to my second ex-wife a number of times since she had to take it under a doctor's order.

Once you start on Coumadin, it is not likely that you will ever get off of it. I wanted no part of it.

*****

I also took Lasix on a daily basis. It was prescribed to counteract the side effects of congestive heart failure (CHF).

Congestive heart failure means that your heart does not beat strongly enough to prevent fluid retention in your body.

With extra fluid in your body, your heart has to work that much harder. It is quite common for post heart-surgery patients to take a diuretic.

A mild case of congestive heart failure is easily managed. Cases of CHF that are more severe require significant medical intervention.

There were days when I did not take my Lasix because I was forgetful. I always knew when I had failed to take it. The swelling in my lower extremities would be noticeable. If I forgot to take it two days in a row, when I resumed the Lasix my weight would drop four or five pounds in one day.

*****

What else was going on?

Well, post-surgically, I was anemic. So I also took over-the-counter iron supplements. In addition, I ate more red meat, raisins and other foods that were rich in iron to elevate my red cell count.

I also watched my calories, my food choices, avoided high-stress situations, and everything else I could think of that might be detrimental while I recovered.

In the meantime, I was all too aware that my depression was masking an anger I felt over the entire situation. But I kept avoiding a confrontation about all of that. I had a full plate to deal with.

*****

With clearance from The Three Wise Men, I had my arthroscopic knee surgery on June 30, 2004. I didn't know it, but my knee looked so bad to Dr. Friedland that he notified Social Security Disability that I should be classified 100% disabled because of my knee. There was not enough cartilage left in the joint in his mind, hence he reported it since he felt I could not rely on it in my work as a claims rep.

I was running out of time on my state disability, having started it in January. It was only good for six months in the State of California.

After an interview with the people at Social Security Disability, and a thorough review of my medical records about my knee, I was formally rated 100% disabled on a permanent basis.

The surgery was at Valleydale Hospital Medical Center. It went smoothly. The "fix" was in once again. Everyone knew who I was and my medical history at the hospital.

Unlike previous arthroscopic surgeries where I had gone home the same day, I stayed overnight after this one. I had all kinds of monitors hooked up to me and a cardiologist in the operating room.

I made it home once again. My activities of daily living were complicated by my recovery from knee surgery.

As if that wasn't enough, I complicated matters further.

*****

I entered into a relationship with a feral, champagne-colored male kitten with medium-length fur. I named him Little Bit. He was a cutie. I fell for him hard.

When I saw him on my front porch screaming his head off for water, he was five weeks old and just a skeleton. I gave him water. Then I went to the store and got Kitten Milk Replacement (KMR). Regular milk would have been too rich for him, and I was not sure if he could eat solid food.

The next morning, he was back at my front door yelling for water and KMR. This time, I took him in the house and gave him food and drink.

I picked him up and saw that he was flea infested and suffered from flea anemia. The fleas were feasting on his blood.

In a few weeks with treatment, he was well. He was a wonderful pet for years.

Caring for him helped me to recover.

*****

My knee rehab was uneventful, which was highly desirable. The post-op pain related to that was negligible compared to the post open-heart-surgery pains. I think that I made it through rehab in eight weeks. The outcome was good, but it wouldn't be the last of my knee troubles. Still, I had negotiated another bump in the road and had my mobility back.

My saving grace for the knee recovery was the fact that I had done a lot of walking and bike riding after the heart surgery. This made my legs very strong when Dr. Friedland operated on me.

I continued to ride my bike for the rest of the summer and beyond. Believe it or not, I even went to Venice Beach to ride several times.

I rode so much that my mountain bike gave up the ghost, and I had to buy a new one. Love those mountain bikes.

*****

In mid-July 2004, I passed the point of no return as far as keeping my job as a Sr. Claims Rep with Farmers Insurance.

Under the Family Medical Leave Act, you got six months off. After that, you could be terminated if you were not ready to return to work.

This was another major stress in my life. I was fifty-five and jobless.

I was offered an opportunity with a different position in another part of Farmers Insurance. However, I was not physically or mentally ready to return to work. What the hell was I going to do for money?

I remained on disability leave as my employer did not press the issue of my returning to work after 6 months.

*****

Late in July 2004, I decided to force the issue regarding my sleep problem. My medical insurance carrier through Farmers said that a sleep study would be covered by my insurance. That was all I needed to hear.

Valleydale Hospital Medical Center had a sleep disorder clinic. So that's where I went.

I met with a neurologist, David Brandeis, MD, who was a UCLA school of medicine alumnus. He ran the clinic. I also met with a nurse who worked for him. We picked a date for the study.

I knew Dr. Brandeis since he had advised my wife for neuro complications from her auto-immune disorder. She had a serious affliction and he helped her a great deal.

*****

On the night of the study, I got to the sleep clinic at the hospital at about 10:00 pm. I was not feeling particularly sleepy as I prepared for the study.

A female tech in the clinic put all kinds of receptors on my head, chest, hands and legs. Then she plugged wire leads to them. The leads ran to an electronic recording device. I think it took her a good half hour to hook me up.

She told me that I would be videotaped as I slept.

I had a difficult time falling asleep that night. After about an hour of restlessness that foreshadowed an eventful night, I went to sleep.

I woke up at about 6:45 am. As soon as the tech saw me rub my eyes awake, she scurried in and hurriedly unhooked me.

She told me that a camera captured the outward manifestations of a sleep disorder related to my PTSD. Apparently, I thrashed wildly in bed flailing my arms and legs, spoke loudly, threw punches and kicks. As she put it, I had been in full bloom. She said it looked and sounded to her like I had been defending myself against some imaginary attackers.

The tech told me that she was sorry I had such a significant sleep disorder and volunteered that the kicks and flailing had frightened her.

*****

On a follow-up visit with Dr. Brandeis, I learned that I did not have a sleep apnea but rather a REM sleep disorder.

The REM part of your sleep cycle is the part where you are in your deepest sleep pattern just before you wake up. He said that I should be considered totally disabled from the sleep disorder. Brandeis said that he viewed the video and that my sleep disorder was very significant. The doctor said that he had a full practice and that he could not take me as a patient.

I thanked him and got copies of the sleep study and filed a new claim with the Department of Veterans Affairs for 100% disability for PTSD. That meant the videotape and results from the monitoring device would be included in my claim.

*****

The powers that be at the Department of Veterans Affairs had been stonewalling me long enough. It was time for them to pay up.

I got a veterans' advocate at the Sepulveda V.A. Medical Center to push my case through. This time, I had it all as far as conclusive evidence to support my position. The veterans' advocate and I worked together, and a week after seeing him, he filed my case and sent the evidence to the Managing Director of the Veteran's Affairs office in Los Angeles.

Dr. Edward Ritvo, a retired psychiatrist who worked for a third party provider reviewing psychiatric claims for disability for the Department of Veterans Affairs, met with me one more time. I gave copies of everything from the sleep study to him.

Ritvo was upset that they had not given me the increase in my disability rating that he felt I should have had eighteen months earlier when he had recommended that. He said that he would write his report in very specific language to get me to 100%.

*****

The medication I started taking shortly after the sleep study (and still take) to control the sleep disorder is Ambien or its generic equivalent, Zolpidem tartrate. It is a powerful medication but it has done wonders for me. I still have nights when 5 O'clock Charlie wakes me up, but they are not too frequent.

I no longer have a lot of incidents where I fight the Vietnam War in my head. That has been a huge relief.

With improved sleep, I began to feel better during the day. My naps became less frequent. I had more energy for life in general.

Before I was prescribed Ambien post-sleep-study, I went on Klonopin very briefly. It was bad news for me as I have described earlier.

I was an old hat at going through the motions to find the right medication for what psychiatric disorder needed to be dealt with. So I gutted it out.

I stayed on Klonopin for only three days before I quit taking it. After that, I returned to see my neurologist so that we could seek another medication for me.

Klonopin is used to treat patients with a history of seizures. It is a heavy duty medication. It does not make you feel like yourself, to say the least, while you're on it. I know that many people have benefitted from using it, but I was not one of them.

I saw an associate of Dr. Brandeis, Lawrence Weinberg, MD, about the Klonopin, and we talked it over. Dr. Weinberg, a highly intelligent yet street-smart neurologist, said that he felt that Ambien would be a better choice than Klonopin. That was after he did a complete neurological work-up on me right on the spot. He didn't miss anything. He was a great doctor. He also read the sleep study report and viewed the videotape.

*****

About two months after submitting my claim in the late fall of 2004, I got the letter from the Department of Veterans Affairs raising my disability rating to 100%. Financially, I dodged a huge bullet once I got the 100% rating from the Department of Veteran's Affairs.

Once it was on the record that I was 100% disabled and required Ambien or its generic equivalent, I got the Department of Veterans Affairs to pay for that medication. They already footed the cost of some other medications that were related to my PTSD.

Being rated 100% disabled by the Department of Veterans Affairs and receiving 100% disability from Social Security for my bad knee were two different ratings by two different agencies.

*****

Collectively, I had dealt with three dragons (knee issues, PTSD, and the heart infection) that had breathed fire trying their best to torch me. I had bobbed and weaved and shucked and jived enough to extinguish them. For three days, I gave myself a respite from everything. I no longer focused on medical problems or anything else. I just sort of let the air out. The three issues had been daunting on their own, let alone together.

Things were ok with me. But they didn't stay that way for long.

I endured a major depressive episode. My nervous breakdown rammed into my brain and consciousness like a speeding 18-wheeler with no brakes.

It was bad, very bad and very difficult to endure. I was fearful that I would get sucked into the vortex of depression and never return. It lasted for a little more than four weeks.

I pulled away from everyone. I didn't put anything important on my plate, as far as decision-making was concerned. My memory was like a kitchen sieve. I was burned out, torched, overwhelmed, sick and tired of feeling sick — not to mention edgy and angry.

My facial expressions gave it all away. There was no mistaking what I was going through if someone looked at my face.

There was no joy, no happiness, and no thoughts about the future or pleasant things. I was in a complete brain fog.

*****

Finally, it started to lift. I was very thankful that I was pulling out of it. With some ups and downs, it passed.

As had been the case with my prior depressive episodes, it was intense but did not last that long. It could have gone on for a long time, but it didn't. My depression ran out of steam.

Shelley was very glad to see me pull out of it. It had concerned her a great deal. I never even flirted with suicidal ideation, but I was royally depressed.

All of it was a reaction to the tough time I had just been through. It was bound to happen and I knew it would. Finally it did. However, the fog blew out of my brain and I was able to think pretty clearly once again.

Part II: My Legal Nightmare

Chapter 10—To Sue or Not to Sue

I was at a fork in the Road of Life about whether or not to sue. Before making a decision about this, some heavy thinking was necessary. I was a decent thinker in my best moments.

Did I have it within me to sue over my MRSA crisis?

I talked to several people about it. The first person I talked to was a former girlfriend who was once a high-school classmate of mine. When I called her, she asked, "To what do I owe the pleasure of your call?" She was sort of half-kidding.

Even though we had broken up several years earlier, I told her what had happened. She couldn't believe it.

She had endured a case of medical malpractice related to a pregnancy. Her decision was to not to file a suit or do anything about it. I wanted her perspective as to why she chose **not** to file suit.

She said that she could not see herself going back through all the hurt she endured. My former girlfriend had debated herself over that decision about three times before she finally let it go. The thought of doing so simply overwhelmed her. Yet she was still scarred emotionally from the negligence.

It was a gut-wrenching story. I listened as she recounted the whole tale one more time and I thanked her for her input. My final thoughts to her included a promise to tell her whichever choice I decided to make.

*****

I spent some time reflecting upon my own situation. The question that I asked was: *Why* **did I want to file a lawsuit?**

My most striking emotion was the anger I felt about the whole incident. I was more pissed off than I had ever been before in my life! As much as I could, I tried to keep it in a bear hug, but sometimes the anger would spill over.

I kept up with regular physical exercise as a way to dissipate the anger.

My psychiatric resident asked me every time I saw him if I was contemplating physical harm to myself or anyone else.

I told him that such thoughts had crossed my mind many times, but that I did not act on those thoughts.

The biggest fear I had was re-living the entire incident if I filed suit. If you think a person's life would be invaded after having open-heart surgery, try going through a lawsuit for damages against someone for medical malpractice. Everything about you is fair game for the other side.

My family members all told me to sue for my injuries.

The decision at hand finally came to me as I had dinner with Shelley, her sister Stephanie, and her brother-in-law Al. As we were about to leave, her sister said, "You know, a little too much happened to you to really let it go. I think you need to tell it to an attorney."

I also thought about the greater good in all of this. There had been obvious administrative lapses within VHMC as far as promptly notifying me. That was intolerable.

Also, doctors who really screw up need to be under a spotlight for what they do or do not do when causing harm to someone. That was absolutely clear in my mind.

I did not relish rehashing the nightmare I had been through. But I eventually I agreed with those who were telling me that it was **too much** to just let it slide.

I realized that I was not in a great mental state when I started my search for an attorney. Yet I took the first few steps anyway. Maybe I could find someone who would help me.

*****

The three defendants in my mind were VHMC, Dr. Morton and Dr. Andrews.

I talked to Shelley since she was a Sr. Legal Secretary in Los Angeles at a large international law firm. She gave me a couple names of attorneys to contact.

The sister of a very well-known medical malpractice plaintiff's attorney worked at Shelley's firm. Her name was Jeannie Brusavich. Her brother's name was Bruce Brusavich.

The first attorney I contacted was Bruce Brusavich. I queried him by mail with a synopsis of my case. He never responded to me. I think I was small potatoes to him.

Additionally, I looked online, in the phone book and even asked for a referral from the San Fernando Valley Bar Association. All in all, I had fifty names to contact as I began my search.

One attorney told me that he only took medical malpractice cases that involved problems during labor and delivery. Another firm said that the medical malpractice cases they took had to be the result of or were caused by a negligent brain injury. Some firms only took medical malpractice cases as a sideline. A few said that they thought what I was alleging would be hard to prove in court after having only a five-minute conversation with me.

"Were they mental?" I wondered.

Several firms admitted that the potential amount of the recovery was too small to interest them. They only wanted cases with larger potential payouts into seven figures.

A couple firms that I called had no idea how a blood infection could damage an aortic valve. They felt that I must have had a congenital defect in that valve that surfaced when I was fifty-five.

I called, mailed and emailed.

*****

Richard T. Lobl of the firm Lobl and Berger in Tarzana, California responded to one of my inquiries. Lobl held a PhD degree as well as a law degree. He had once been an instructor at the UCLA School of Medicine. I saw an ad for his firm in the yellow pages.

We spoke to each other over the phone and I learned that he had been a practicing attorney specializing in medical malpractice cases for a number of years. Lobl said that as long as the case had the potential for monetary damages, he was interested.

I briefly explained the circumstances of the case to him. He asked me a few questions. We talked for about fifteen minutes during that first phone conversation. Finally, we agreed to meet.

I agreed to provide names, addresses and phone numbers of all possible defendants in the case. I also had to obtain copies of all the medical records relating to my treatment, diagnosis and care (or lack of it) from March through April 2004.

Lobl told me that he would get back to me within a few weeks. He was headed for a much needed vacation and, after that, he would need a week to look at everything. He told me to get a copy of all medical records from the hospital and Dr. Andrews which I did.

At least someone was interested enough in my case to take a hard look at it. That was a positive sign for me. Also, if I needed to file a lawsuit, it would be well within a year of the incident itself or one year since the discovery of any damages I suffered as a result of negligence medical malpractice.

Two weeks later, I dropped off all the materials that Lobl requested. The following week, Lobl called to say that he wanted me to meet him in his office to discuss the merits of my case.

*****

Rick Lobl's office did not have an aura of affluence. It was neat, clean and functional. The furniture was ok but not highbrow. The office was fitting for the kind of office building he leased space in. It was just a suite in an office building. There was nothing memorable about the suite or the office building.

Rick Lobl looked like a college professor with his facial hair and glasses. He was at least forty pounds overweight.

His hair was graying; he was bespectacled and sported a beard and a mustache. He was a 50-something guy, over 6' tall and had a relaxed, yet commanding voice. Lobl exuded confidence.

"Your case is worth pursuing. Yes, there was negligence malpractice by three parties," he told me. "Your case meets all the criteria of the malpractice laws here in California. The records I reviewed from the ER group, the hospital and Dr. Andrews show what did and didn't happen very clearly. The surgery you had could have been avoided. There is no question about that."

I asked, "Have you ever had a case like this?"

"Yes. It was a few years ago. It also involved a blood infection that was misdiagnosed to the detriment of the patient. We prevailed at trial."

"It's hard for me to take that the surgery could have been avoided." I covered my face with both hands as I took his words in.

"I would estimate that your case is worth about half a million dollars. It's not a huge case but it is worth pursuing."

"What seems to be the key point of contention if there is one?"

"Looks like the defense might argue that the infection was beyond 'the point of no return' when the blood culture and sensitivity were ordered," Lobl said.

"Sensitivity...?"

"To certain antibiotics. Not every antibiotic will treat every infection."

That was the first time I was made aware of the sensitivity an infection could have to certain kinds of drugs even though I discussed it earlier in the book.

I repeated what Dr. Morton had told me about Augmentin; that is, that this drug would "**take care of any infection**" I had.

"Well, he got it wrong. Lucky for you that you went back to the ER on April 12th. You were running out of time. I'm guessing maybe four days at the most until death was a high probability. You had a one centimeter infection on your heart valve. At three centimeters, they cut you open — STAT."

That was the first I had ever heard about that scenario.

I was convinced that Lobl had read my records and in some detail. He mentioned other points that reinforced that notion. Lobl also displayed an understanding of the pathology of the infection that almost killed me.

"It's a textbook case of how infectious bacterial endocarditis manifests itself," he said.

Rick Lobl revealed to me that he knew an ER doctor named Ed Morton. Dr. Morton had been an expert witness for Lobl's client in a case Lobl had won. Dr. Morton testified under oath. Lobl gave me a few of the details about the case and Morton's testimony. The true significance of this did not register with me at that moment.

"The guy was really good," Lobl offered.

I got a puzzled look on my face.

"Mr. Lobl, one of the potential defendants in this case is an ER doctor at Valleydale Hospital named Morton."

"It couldn't be the same guy..."

Lobl pulled out a personal phone book. He searched through it. Then he punched in a number, the number of Edward Nathan Morton, MD.

"Dr. Morton, please."

I waited for the other shoe to drop.

Lobl said, "Dr. Morton, this is Rick Lobl."

After two minutes of small talk, Lobl told him why he had called. He advised Dr. Morton that he could be named as a defendant in a medical malpractice case that would also involve Valleydale Hospital Medical Center and Raymond Andrews, MD. Lobl gave Morton some background and told him that the case would be about negligence malpractice.

I picked up on the fact that Morton remembered me as a patient and that he had gotten in trouble over his handling of my case once I was admitted to VHMC.

The two of them talked for maybe five more minutes before they said their good-byes.

Lobl told me that Dr. Morton asked Lobl to keep him out of the lawsuit. I was told that Morton said that he would help Lobl go after the hospital. Dr. Morton added that he would use his influence to make the hospital understand that they were negligent in this case since the hospital lab results were not communicated to me in a timely manner. Because of that, the infection went bonkers.

Lobl said that Morton told him he would have no problem being named in the suit. He told Lobl that if he had liability in this case, he would settle out of court. He also told Rick that it was ok with him if Lobl was my attorney against him.

Lobl sat in his chair grinning from ear to ear like a Cheshire cat. He was beaming.

A moment later, he launched into a discourse about how he ran his law practice against defendants and their respective malpractice insurance carriers. He said that he had a routine and that he didn't vary from it. Lobl said that he handled all of his cases the same way.

He made it very clear that in his practice he saw the same defendants over and over, and that he saw the same medical malpractice insurance carriers over and over, and the same law firms over and over. Lobl said that the same lawyers defended the same defendants for the same insurance companies.

Lobl told me that he didn't show anger to the defendants or their insurance companies about what had happened to his clients.

In short, he wanted me to know that he fished in the same pond over and over and that he wasn't going to rock the boat on the waters where he made his living.

Lobl used the term "closed club." He said that this meant that everyone in the medical malpractice arena knew who the "players" were. He noted that there was mutual respect and that this was the way he handled medical malpractice cases.

He further offered that yelling and screaming at defendants and their carriers was out. Lobl wanted no drama that way. He said that if I became his client, he would expect me to behave the same way. No yelling and screaming, no matter what they said about me or what they might allude to.

I got a strong feeling that Richard T. Lobl was a control freak. He would go to the nth degree to avoid muddying the waters in his pond.

My brain was in a half-fog the day that I sat in Lobl's office. I was seeking someone to help me and I was not thinking 100% clearly. Several important inferences that he made didn't sink in. I wouldn't figure them out until much, much later.

Should I have believed Mr. Lobl?

For one thing, I had no input about my case from any other plaintiff's malpractice attorney. With no firsthand knowledge of the unwritten rules of medical malpractice cases that he offered up, I believed him. I was outside of my element and uncomfortable, yet I knew that I wanted to file a lawsuit.

Lobl gave me a client retainer agreement form as we talked. The agreement detailed what he and I would agree to do if he handled my case.

Once home, I felt relieved knowing that someone would take my case. The conversation between Lobl and Morton troubled me. Still, I surmised that I was facing a legal maze that I could not navigate alone and that I had the opportunity to hire an attorney very experienced at navigating the legal waters ahead.

*****

Who would you call for background information regarding a medical/legal situation like mine?

I called my first ex-wife Wendy. I had a long conversation with her about Rick Lobl.

She said that he had an ongoing case against her firm involving negligence in a nursing home. My ex said that he seemed to be a real tiger. According to her, Lobl had appealed the case twice in seeking a plaintiff's verdict for his client. She said that he seemed competent in a court room and that he was well-spoken.

Her assessment of Lobl was a major reason I chose to retain him as my attorney.

*****

The next morning, after talking to Shelley, my brother, and my children Darrell, Melinda, and Jessica, I signed the papers to have Lobl handle my case. I drove straight to his office and dropped them off.

With little fanfare, I started on an "E ticket" ride through the medical malpractice court system. I had no clue as to what awaited me. There was no hint of what I would be subjected to by both sides as the major players went about their business. To them, it was business and to me, it was about my life.

I called my ex-girlfriend and told her that I was going to file a lawsuit. She said, "You have a lot more guts than I did."

Chapter 11—Let the Prelims Begin

Do the Marquis of Queensbury rules of boxing apply to a medical malpractice lawsuit in California?

*****

In California, medical malpractice lawsuits are covered by The MICRA (Medical Injury Compensation Reform Act of 1975). Essentially, it has remained the same as it was the day it was enacted.

This law was meant to protect physicians and their medical malpractice insurance companies with very little thought given to injured plaintiffs comparably speaking. By imposing limits on non-economic damages (commonly known as "pain and suffering"), it was hoped that all physicians could find affordable coverage in a time of rapidly rising med mal insurance premiums.

The only benefit to consumers was that this would provide a guaranteed way to sue for damages and collect money with a favorable settlement or verdict. The alternative was trying to collect from an uninsured physician or medical practitioner who had no money to pay out of pocket.

*****

On Monday August 2, 2004, in keeping with the law under section 364.1 of the *California Code of Civil Procedure*, copies of the "90-Day Notice of Intent to Commence Action" letters were mailed to: Valleydale Hospital Medical Center; Valleydale Emergency Medical Group; Edward Nathan Morton, MD; Raymond Andrews, MD; William Kent, P.A.; and they were also sent to The Complaint Unit of the Medical Board of California. At that point, a civil lawsuit was prepared.

After the suit was filed on August 12, 2004 in (the Chatsworth, California) Superior Court of the County of Los Angeles **known as *David Folck vs. Valleydale Hospital Medical Center, et al.*,** both sides entered into the discovery phase of the case. When the suit was filed initially, Dr. Andrews was not named as a defendant.

The suit alleged that:

"On or about March 28, 2004, and continuing thereafter, during the course of the care, hospital admission, surgery and post-surgical care, the defendants, and each of them, so negligently, wrongfully, carelessly, recklessly diagnosed, failed to monitor, failed to inform plaintiff of a positive culture and sensitivity, failed to provide appropriate antibiotics, failed to refer plaintiff to a specialist, such that plaintiff developed vegetation on his heart valve, thereby causing permanent injury to his heart and body."

Once a medical malpractice case is filed, defendant malpractice insurance companies select the law firms that they want to represent their clients. Patient records are obtained and reviewed on both sides. Experts are employed to review the records in detail. The experts form opinions about the case in their respective areas of expertise. Results and opinions are sent to the respective sides. After that, depositions are scheduled for all of the people who might have pertinent information about the case. In my case, these included a ward clerk, several doctors, experts in various specialties including medical specialties, and that of yours truly.

In the practice and custom of law in the United State of America, a deposition is a written record from out-of-court sworn oral testimony by a witness. It is used for discovery or later at a trial. Depositions are commonly used in litigation and are most always taken outside of a court of law. A judge is usually not present. Lawyers for opposing sides conduct depositions.

Litigants use depositions as part of the discovery process in gathering evidence before a trial. Commonly, a paid, licensed court reporter is used to take down every word that is spoken on the record. In some legal jurisdictions, a written affidavit will suffice. Specific instructions are given at the beginning and immediately before the end of a deposition.

Discovery means, basically, or is supposed to mean "You show me yours (evidence) and I'll show you mine (evidence)."

Excerpts from some of the depositions follow. Only excerpts are included because the number of pages of sworn, deposed testimony numbers in the hundreds. Including everything that was said would be repetitive and boring. No thought was given to censoring any person who was deposed by including excerpts only and ignoring some people completely. I tried to include only the main evidence from the depositions in the interest of brevity.

Why did I include deposition testimony?

What gets said for real and what gets said in a deposition are not necessarily the same. In other words, the truth can be stretched or lies told about what really happened during a deposition.

Also, if you saw what I saw, it would give you the same feeling for the case that I had. I'm asking you to look at it through my eyes.

To some who are sworn, telling "the truth" has no meaning. They avoid it to save their reputations. Or they shade it for the same reason. Some flat out lie.

For defendants (including their medical malpractice insurance carriers), their desire is to be dropped from the lawsuit or, if a judgment is rendered for the plaintiff, they want to minimize the financial exposure.

DEPOSITION OF DAVID LEWIS FOLCK

My deposition was taken on Wednesday January 12, 2005 at the offices of Lobl and Berger in Tarzana, California. Present were court reporter Janice C. Watkins, Christopher Wright representing VHMC, Jennifer Renaud representing the Valleydale Emergency Medical Group, and Linda K. Rurangirwa representing Dr. Andrews. Michael Berger represented me.

Mr. Wright: And I understand you're probably taking some medications. Does any of that affect your ability to remember things or—

Mr. Folck: No.

Mr. Wright: —answer questions? Ok. Good.

Mr. Folck: No.

146

Mr. Wright: Anybody in your family have any medical training?

Mr. Berger: You mean his immediate family?

Mr. Wright: Yeah, immediate family.

Mr. Folck: My mother was a registered nurse.

Mr. Wright: Before March 2004, did you ever have any heart problems?

Mr. Berger: Well, the question is vague and ambiguous as phrased. Also calls for speculation, but you can go ahead and answer if you understand.

Mr. Folck: No.

Mr. Wright: Do you know if anyone in your family has ever had any heart disease or heart surgery?

Mr. Folck: Yes.

Mr. Wright: Who is that?

Mr. Folck: My mother.

Mr. Wright: Do you know what the condition was?

Mr. Folck: Arterial blockage.

Mr. Wright: Do you know what surgery she had?

Mr. Folck: Bypass operation.

Mr. Wright: How long have you been treating with Dr. Amico?

Mr. Folck: Since April 12, 2004.

Mr. Wright: Is he your primary-care doctor?

Mr. Folck: Yes.

Mr. Wright: Who was your primary-care doctor before him?

Mr. Folck: Dr. Raymond Andrews.

Mr. Wright: Ok. What prompted you to change doctors?

Mr. Folck: After this incident, there was *no doubt* (that) I was going to change doctors.

Mr. Wright: Other than Dr. Amico, have any other doctors said you will need future care, future medical care?

Mr. Folck: Yes.

Mr. Wright: Which doctors?

Mr. Folck: Dr. Schwinger.

Mr. Wright: And what has he said in that regard?

I told those present that Dr. Schwinger told me that I would need future office visits, future EKGs, future echocardiograms, medications, blood tests, x-rays, etc. Continuing on, I told him that Dr. Schwinger told me that I would probably need another open-heart surgery in ten years. I also told him that Dr. Soltero concurred with Dr. Schwinger about the medical care I would need and a future open-heart surgery.

Mr. Wright: Ok. Why did you go to the Emergency Room on April 6th?

Mr. Folck: My high fevers were persisting.

Mr. Wright: When you say, "high fever," did high fevers, was your fever going up and down? I mean temperature?

Mr. Folck: I could have a high fever for several hours in a row before it broke.

I told those present about my first visit to Dr. Andrews' office after my first visit to the ER and that my complaints were persistent fever, and a respiratory problem, specifically a cough with some production. I told them that Andrews prescribed Biaxcin. Continuing, I told them that Dr. Andrews was treating me for bronchitis.

I told them about my second office visit with Dr. Andrews on April 6th. I told them that my chief complaint was my persistent intermittent fever

148

and the respiratory problems. My testimony included that Dr. Andrews switched me to Augmentin. I told them that Dr. Andrews was sticking to his diagnosis of bronchitis.

Mr. Wright: Did he (Andrews) recommend that you go to the Emergency Room?

Mr. Folck: Yes.

Mr. Wright: So, when you went to the Emergency Room later that day then, did you have any additional symptoms?

Mr. Folck: The same symptoms persisted, a high fever, the respiratory problem, I felt weak, I was miserable.

Mr. Wright: Were your symptoms worsening?

Mr. Folck: They were worsening.

I told them all that I had taken my own temperature at home that afternoon and it had registered 102.9 on my thermometer.

Mr. Wright: But what was the lower range?

Mr. Folck: 100.

Mr. Wright: Do you remember how many times you were taking your temperature per day?

Mr. Folck: Three or four times a day.

Mr. Wright: Did he (Morton) look at you; did he provide you with a diagnosis?

Mr. Folck: He did look at me for the respiratory problem and the fever.

I also told Wright that, at the ER, Dr. Morton concurred with Dr. Andrews' diagnosis after I told Morton what Dr. Andrews had told me. I told them that he also concurred with the prescription for Augmentin that Dr. Andrews prescribed earlier in the day.

Mr. Wright: Do you remember speaking with Dr. Fujita on April 6th?

Mr. Folck: No.

Mr. Wright: Do you even know Dr. Fujita?

Mr. Folck: I don't recall speaking to him, no.

Mr. Wright: Ok. Do you know if you were ever treated by someone named Dr. Fujita at any time?

Mr. Folck: I can't recall.

I simply could not remember my brief interaction with Dr. Fujita. Then, under additional questioning, I told all present that I saw Dr. Andrews on April 9th presenting the same symptoms to him: continuing high fevers, continuing respiratory complaints, and a cough.

Mr. Wright: What did Dr. Andrews tell you to do, if anything?

Mr. Folck: Continue with Augmentin to treat both conditions.

Mr. Wright: Why did you go to the Emergency Room on April 12th?

Mr. Folck: I was very sick from the fever and the respiratory problem. They were both worsening.

Mr. Wright: Had you coughed up blood at any point?

Mr. Folck: Earlier in the day on the 12th of April 2004.

Mr. Wright: Did any of those doctors (Amico, Soltero, Schwinger, Kuhlman) tell you how you came to have vegetation on your heart?

Mr. Folck: Yes.

Mr. Wright: Who said what?

Mr. Folck: Each of them indicated that the problem with my heart valve was an undiagnosed, untreated *staphylococcus (aureus)* infection.

Mr. Wright: Do you recall, what, if any, future ailments you were informed of that might arise if you didn't go forward with the valve replacement surgery?

150

Mr. Folck: Yes.

Mr. Wright: What were you told?

Mr. Folck: Certainly I'd be at risk for further heart problems.

Mr. Berger: Was the doctor specific?

Mr. Folck: Including heart attacks which could be fatal.

I told all present that Dr. Soltero advised me that it would be likely that I would need additional valve replacement surgeries beyond this one. And that he told me the surgery itself could be risky due to unforeseen consequences and that I could die during surgery. He also advised me that I might need a pacemaker in the future.

Mr. Wright: What did he (Dr. Soltero) tell you about the prognosis after surgery or anything about the surgery?

Mr. Folck: He said that the surgery had gone well. Soltero said I would be kept in intensive care for as long as necessary. If my condition improved, they would move me out of intensive care.

I told everyone in the room that after the surgery, my fever and respiratory problems improved. Continuing, I said that they had shown improvement before the surgery after I was admitted on April 12th.

I told them that I had asked Dr. Andrews for a stronger antibiotic on April 10th, and that he had switched me to Levaquin.

Mr. Wright: At any point after March 28th, 2004, did anybody other than your counsel or any doctors communicate to you the results of the blood culture and sensitivity that was taken that day?

Mr. Folck: Yes.

Mr. Wright: And when was that?

Mr. Folck: April 6th.

Mr. Wright: And who told you that?

Mr. Folck: Dr. Harold Morton.

151

Mr. Wright: And what did he say?

Mr. Folck: He said I had tested positive for *staphylococcus (aureus)* infection in my blood culture.

In my previous remembrance, I did not completely recall what Dr. Morton had told me. In reality, I didn't know *Staphylococcus* from *Streptococcus*.

Mr. Berger: What else, if anything did the doctor tell you at that time?

Mr. Folck: He concurred with Dr. Andrews' prescription of Augmentin and told me that the **Augmentin would take care of _any_ infection I had.**

The room was silent. Mr. Berger nodded his head up and down once after I had said those fateful words. When no one spoke, the court reporter looked at me and shook her head back and forth.

At that point, Mr. Wright became quite flustered.

The stress of re-living the entire affair started getting to me. Intellectually, I knew that Mr. Wright and the other attorneys needed to question me some more. But I was goddamn sick of it all.

I told them that the results of the blood culture and sensitivity were communicated to me on April 12th by the ER doctor and the three doctors who I saw upstairs.

As I responded to more questions, I told them that other than Dr. Morton and the other doctors I mentioned, no one ever communicated the results to me. Then I recalled my interaction with Dr. Morton on April 6th.

Mr. Folck: He (Morton) was looking at a clipboard. He said to me that a clerk in the ER had called my home phone number, but had reached a Spanish-speaking person. He further asked me if my phone number was 818-xxx-xxxx and I said it was.

I added that the number he asked me about was my home phone number, and that I had no Spanish-speaking people in my household and that I lived alone.

I explained, very carefully, that all three of the doctors I saw after being admitted said that if my infection had been diagnosed properly, with timely notification and managed as it should have been according to the standard of medical care for such cases, **that the open-heart surgery would have been unnecessary.**

There was some questioning about my current employment situation, and I told them that I was not working and didn't know when I would be working. All of this was very distasteful to deal with since not working was a huge sore spot with me.

Jennifer Renaud (representing the Valleydale Emergency Medical Group) asked me if I had had any other medical issues subsequent to the surgery.

I said that I had had to recover from the heart surgery and then had an arthroscopic knee surgery including rehab for both. As I answered more questions, I revealed that I had been overnight at Valleydale Hospital Medical Center for a sleep study. And that the study found that I had a significant REM sleep disorder. I also told them I was taking Ambien on a daily basis for the sleep disorder at present.

I was close to a breaking point with all the questioning and probing and the general direction of the deposition. I wanted to leave and go for a long solitary bike ride.

Finally, we took a break.

After going back on the record, Ms. Renaud went through a detailed inquiry into my visits and treatment from the V.A. It felt like "piling on" to me. I had already explained in detail through the answers to pre-deposition questions about why I was treated by the V.A., when I first went there ad nauseum.

It was bad enough that I had to talk about the whole infection debacle. Talking about the PTSD stuff drained me even more and made me feel edgy.

I explained in detail how my sleep was torched, why it was torched, how my depression was heightened, why it was heightened and on and on. As questioning continued, I said that I had had all the symptoms I was complaining about on prior occasions but that they were worse as the after effects of the surgery hit me.

Ms. Renaud rehashed old testimony that I had previously answered as if she had been asleep when I testified about the subjects she wanted to cover. I thought that she was "mental."

Linda Rurangirwa (representing Dr. Andrews) took over the questioning. Again, a lot of the same old stuff.

It occurred to me that attorneys had to show how they were spending their clients' money by asking so many duplicate questions. You know, justifying their existence.

Ms. Rurangirwa asked me everything under the sun about my visits with Dr. Andrews and my phone call with him on April 10th. Talk about being anal. She was that in her questioning.

I was getting dizzy from all the questions. My concentration was waning and heading south.

To clarify one of Ms. Rurangirwa's questions, Mr. Berger interceded.

Mr. Berger: She wants to know if Dr. Andrews did in fact tell you on the evening of April 10th during this phone conversation to go to the Emergency Room; did you in fact go to the Emergency Room? And, if not, was there a reason that you did not go to the Emergency Room per Dr. Andrews' instructions or recommendations.

Mr. Folck: No, I did not go.

Mr. Berger: And she wants to know—

Mr. Folck: I felt very weak. I was extremely tired from more than two weeks of very poor sleep, and I'll let it stand at that.

Ms. Rurangirwa: Did you ask anybody if they would be able to take you to the Emergency Room on April 10th, 2004?

Mr. Folck: No.

After that, I went over the phone number story with Mr. Wright. I told him that I received other phone calls on or about April 30th, the date that the blood culture results were known. Under additional questioning, I added that I did not receive any phone calls from anyone at VHMC.

I felt like a "Looney Tunes" character.

Ms. Rurangirwa: And has your heart surgery prevented you from seeking other employment?

I paused a long time. I could feel the tears welling up with all the hurt and anger behind them. Then I let her have it.

Mr. Folck: Frankly, I've been too goddamn depressed about the whole thing!

A moment later, with my head buried in my chest, **I cried a waterfall of tears.**

Mr. Berger: You need to take a break?

Mr. Folck: I'm ok.

Mr. Berger: Ok, let's take a break.

I remember walking out of the room and I wanted to yell, "She is an idiot, a damn idiot with a law degree. What the hell does she think — that I'm just going to ditty bop out and slide into a new job?" But I didn't. Mr. Berger had advised me not to lose my temper.

I went into another room and cried and ranted for about ten minutes loud enough to be heard in outer space.

Then I collected myself, drank some water, and went back into the conference room where the deposition was being taken.

As I sat there, I fixed my gaze on Ms. Rurangirwa with an angry stare. My nostrils flared. She turned away. Then she caught my gaze again and turned away again.

We went back on the record.

155

Ms. Rurangirwa: I just have a couple of more questions. You stated that you were treating with Dr. Weinberg, a neurologist. Since October or November of 2004, have any of your visits to Dr. Weinberg — are any of those related to any of the damages or injuries that you're claiming in this lawsuit?

From then on to the end of the deposition, I spoke with my teeth clenched in a very angry deep tone of voice.

Mr. Folck: Yes.

Ms. Rurangirwa: How many of those visits were related to it?

I leaned a little closer to her direction.

Mr. Folck: All of them!

I wanted to show her how pissed I was at her.

Ms. Rurangirwa: And what was the purpose of those visits?

I put my right thumb and index finger to the bridge of my nose, lowered my head, and shook it side to side and then I spoke.

Mr. Folck: For treatment of a REM sleep disorder!

At that point, I wanted to say to her, "I'm still seeing him because I knew I would get brain damage from talking to an attorney like you and I was right!" But I didn't.

Finally, it ended. I quickly got to my feet and headed out of the room in a big hurry without speaking to any of the attorneys.

After that, I had a brief meeting with Michael Berger to the effect that I had done well and that he was sorry that the questions and answers were so painful. I felt as though I wanted to kill Linda Rurangirwa.

DEPOSITION OF EDWARD NATHAN MORTON, MD

On Wednesday March 2, 2005, Dr. Morton was deposed in Los Angeles by my attorney, Rick Lobl. Also present were court reporter Susan Ann

Graham, and attorneys Patricia Daehnke (Dr. Andrews), Richard Ryan (Dr. Morton), and Sara Clark (VHMC).

Prior to attending medical school, Edward Nathan Morton once worked as a research engineer. Morton held a BS in aeronautical engineering from a prominent Midwestern university. After that, he obtained an MS in Engineering from a Southern university.

In 1981, he obtained a Doctor of Medicine, MD degree from a Southern medical school. He completed a residency in Emergency Medicine at Los Angeles County USC Medical Center in 1984.

Morton obtained his license to practice medicine in California in 1982. He was board certified in Emergency Medicine in 1989 and re-certified in 1999.

Basically, Rick Lobl followed a timeline of my interactions with Dr. Morton and others working in the VHMC Emergency Room from March 28, 2004 through April 6, 2004.

To start things off, Dr. Morton said that Dr. Friedland called him on March 28th and asked him to see me in the ER.

Dr. Morton: He (Folck) had a fever and swelling of his right knee and (Friedland) asked me to tap his knee and get cultures and **I did a CBC and a blood culture** and to call him back with the results. Dr. Friedland did my mother's hip on Christmas Day (2003) when she fell in my home, so I know Jerry (Friedland) very well.

Morton looked at the documents related to my visit that day and noted what I had told the triage nurse.

Dr. Morton: Complains of right knee swelling, weakness and fever.

Dr. Morton read from the triage notes that my fever that day was 99.4 orally and that I had complained of fever as high as 102.4. Referring to his notes, he indicated that I had a swollen right knee with no evidence of any redness or red streaks (which might indicate the presence of infection) or anything. He said that my knee did not feel "hot" to him like you might find from gout or an infectious type knee. Dr. Morton indicated all of those things in his written notes.

Morton said that there was nothing from the preliminary blood results that indicated anything to be concerned about as far as an infection. He noted that he drained my right knee of 60 ccs of knee joint fluid and another 40 ccs of slightly bloody knee joint fluid.

He said that he had called Dr. Friedland back.

Dr. Morton: I have tapped his knee, it does not look hot. It is not warm. I don't think that his fever has anything to do with his knee tap.

Mr. Lobl: And my understanding is at the same time you drew the CBC you had some of that sent for a culture and sensitivity, is that correct?

Dr. Morton: Yes, sir.

Mr. Lobl: And what was your purpose in doing that?

Dr. Morton: Dr. Friedland asked that I do that.

Mr. Lobl: Under clinical impression, you have written right knee effusion secondary to arthritis; is that correct?

Dr. Morton: Yes.

Mr. Lobl: Then it says fever secondary to viral illness. What is the basis of that opinion?

Dr. Morton: Well, I didn't have any basis for any other reason that the patient would have a fever. I mean, he wasn't coughing. I didn't see any other source.

Mr. Lobl: But at the same time you did withdraw and send some blood for culture and sensitivity?

Dr. Morton: Yes. **I think that was because of what Dr. Friedland wanted**. It would not have been something I would have done based upon this patient's presentation there.

Yet, on the notes he wrote from the visit, there was no notation of Dr. Friedland mentioning that to him. Dr. Friedland's request for a blood culture was nowhere on the triage notes.

I presented 101.7 as my fever about forty minutes after being admitted at 5:50 pm when I was examined by Dr. Morton. Morton indicated that I had been given Tylenol.

The knee joint fluid came back negative for any infection. The same could not be said of the blood culture, according to Morton.

On Tuesday March 30, 2004, a female hospital ward clerk named Bina Sehmi spoke to Dr. Morton and told him that she had a report that Mr. Folck had tested positive for infection on his blood culture. Morton indicated that it was customary to notify the originating physician or one of the physicians on duty of any "positive for infection" reports. He was unsure whether the report indicated sensitivity of my infection to any particular medications.

It was at this point that Dr. Morton interjected that a positive result on a blood culture for infection could in fact be a **false positive.**

Next Dr. Morton indicated that he verbally informed Dr. Friedland of my positive blood culture when Friedland entered the Emergency Room about twenty minutes after Bina told Dr. Morton of my blood culture report results.

Dr. Morton: Jerry, that patient that I tapped the knee on the other night, he has a positive blood culture and we tried to call him, but we cannot get through with the number we have. So Jerry sat down at the desk and called his office to see what number they had, and I don't know if he gave us a different number or it was the same number.

Mr. Lobl: Do you have any recollection that Bina told you what happened when she attempted to call the number that she believed was Mr. Folck's?

Dr. Morton: It seems, the best I can remember, that she called a couple of times before Dr. Friedland got there and either we got no answer or a wrong number or we got somebody who spoke in Spanish, and I didn't recall if that was exactly — if that was right after we spoke with Jerry or not, but I know there was one number we called that didn't seem to work and another we called and we had somebody answer in Spanish.

Mr. Lobl: What happened after that relative to trying to get a hold of Mr. Folck?

Dr. Morton: Well, I told Bina, I said we need to follow up on this patient, you know, and make sure he is contacted, and she said she would take care of it, whatever they do, send out a telegram or send out a registered letter and try and call the patient's physician if we can find out who it is, and on the chart all we had was Dr. Friedland, I think, so I don't know if at that time who else he was seeking as a physician.

Mr. Lobl: But there was no specific statement as to who of the two of you would be following him (Folck)?

Dr. Morton: No. He didn't say, "Look, I will take care of it," you know, or I didn't say, "Jerry, don't worry about it, we will take care of it." There was never that kind of discussion.

Dr. Morton stated that he never had any further discussions with Bina about any additional follow-up she had trying to reach me. Dr. Morton also stated that he did not know of any specific mechanism to contact a patient with a positive blood culture beyond phone calls. He said that they probably existed, but that he did not know what they were specifically. Morton also stated that he did not know or could not recall any other cases where notification of a patient was a problem.

Morton said that probably the reason William Kent, P.A., who treated me for my wrist problem, didn't have my chart showing previous visits was that it was 4 o'clock in the morning when I was there and that no one was asked to go and get my chart. He said that he believed that the person who would have been available to do that was the night nursing supervisor. At that time, x-ray records were available on the computer system, but not past patient charts.

The questioning moved ahead to Tuesday April 6, 2004.

Mr. Lobl: All right. And tell me, if you can, what happened on that date. How were you first notified he (Folck) was here?

Basically, the story was that I was in the ER for intermittent fever times nine days. I was assigned to Dr. Ron Fujita, a second-year resident in the family practice residency program. Morton was supervising Ron Fujita. Fujita asked him what to do.

Morton said that he remembered my name as someone who the Emergency Room had been trying to get a hold of. He said that he told Dr.

Fujita that I had shown abnormal results on some lab work and that they needed to call my current physician and discuss the necessary follow-up for me.

Dr. Morton: I believe I said to him (Folck), "We have been trying to call you and we don't have the right number," and, you know, I don't remember any other details like, you know, you have an infected blood culture or infected knee or anything like that. I don't recall that. But I do remember going in and talking to him and saying that we had been trying to call him.

He later added that he said they had been trying to call me about my blood work. Again, Dr. Morton said that he didn't remember if he said anything about any positive blood culture result for infection on my blood culture.

Morton said that when he talked to me on the 6th, he had no knowledge of whether or not I was ultimately contacted about the lab results prior to April 6th. He also said that I seemed surprised that no one had been able to reach me.

Dr. Morton: Nobody ever said, "Oh, my doctor knows the results." It was definitely never said that definitely he knew the results or that his doctor knew the results.

Morton said that Fujita told him (Morton) that he called and spoke with Dr. Andrews and gave him the results. He said that he, Morton, never spoke to Dr. Andrews and that the person who did that was Dr. Fujita.

Dr. Morton: Well, I asked him later after I heard about the lawsuit, I said, "Ron, did you ever discuss the blood cultures with Dr. Andrews?" And he said, "Yes, I told him the blood cultures and sensitivities." And I also asked him did he ever discuss those results with me about the positive blood culture, and he said no.

Dr. Morton acknowledged that he knew the lab results on the 30th but denied 100% knowledge that it was *staph*, and also that he did not know if it was a true positive result but perhaps a false positive. He said that by having Dr. Fujita call Dr. Andrews and notify him of the blood culture results and the sensitivities to certain antibiotics that the responsibilities of the Emergency Department as far as notifying me had been fulfilled.

On one portion of my chart, Dr. Fujita entered, "Discussed with Dr. Andrews. Patient stable. Continue Augmentin. Follow up Friday." Following

161

that entry, there was an entry that read, "Concur with resident's disposition, discussed with Dr. Andrews. Patient has prescription from primary doctor for Augmentin and he was sent home."

When asked what he thought the Augmentin was for, Dr. Morton said he believed that it was for pneumonia.

Mr. Lobl: Did the culture and sensitivity show the bacteria to be sensitive (resistant) to Augmentin?

Dr. Morton: Well, it doesn't state Augmentin specifically; it has several different drugs. It doesn't say Augmentin specifically.

Mr. Lobl: Is Augmentin in the same class as one of the other medications that is listed?

Dr. Morton: Yes.

Mr. Lobl: Which one?

Dr. Morton: Penicillin.

Mr. Lobl: And penicillin is a resistant strain?

Dr. Morton: That is correct.

Mr. Lobl: And so penicillin would not have been the medication of choice for this particular *staph*?

Dr. Morton: That is correct.

Morton said that there was confusion about the color of the lab report that Dr. Fujita had handed him — it was white and not blue and it was unfamiliar to Dr. Morton.

Dr. Morton: So I basically flipped back through and just picked out the blue paper, which was the lab results, and that is what I recorded on my chart. **So I missed this sensitivity report because it was printed on white paper. I didn't look for that specifically.** I think the natural response when you get sued is, as you know, you are upset, you are frustrated, and I was frustrated probably with so many people (who) had touched this chart or this patient and the patient never, you know, got treated appropriately, and I think I was frustrated with that whole mechanism. You know, his orthopedist knew it, his internist probably knew it maybe before, but certainly after he had been to the ER the second time when I was there, and you just get frustrated, how does this happen? Where did the mechanism go wrong? Where did the system fail? I think it was the kind of generic frustration, you know, there is something wrong here, why can't we — how can we fix this or why did this happen, you know.

After that, Mr. Ryan instructed Dr. Morton not to answer several of Mr. Lobl's questions.

Dr. Morton said that he never heard Dr. Ron Fujita discuss any of the lab results or sensitivities with Dr. Andrews.

*****

In reading the transcript of Dr. Morton, I felt that he answered nervously, that he was purposely vague on a number of answers, that he showed an "It's not my problem" attitude about the whole lack of timely notification and the failure in not picking up the sensitivity (resistance) of my blood culture to any penicillin-based drug. He was dancing as fast as he could. His statement near the end of the deposition about his frustration was pure whitewash. Morton had failed miserably as a doctor for his part in my medical debacle. It didn't take a rocket scientist to see that, either.

Several practicing physicians told me that no good doctor ever addresses a patient's condition as if the reading of a lab result could be a false positive. They said a good doctor *always* considers that a lab result that is positive really is positive. Yet Dr. Morton tried to advance the false positive idea.

Several practicing physicians told me that no good doctor would ever let a patient go back out into the world on the wrong antibiotic. Dr. Morton knew that I had a *Staphylococcus aureus* blood infection, which also meant that there was the possibility that it was a MRSA infection. Because of that, he needed to be damn sure of the sensitivity of the blood culture to certain antibiotics, yet he just acted so capriciously and ignored that possibility.

DEPOSITION OF RAYMOND ARTHUR ANDREWS, MD

Dr. Andrews was deposed on Friday March 11, 2005 at the law offices of Lobl and Berger. The court reporter was Stephanie L. Faas. Also present were: Michael Berger, Christopher Wright for Valleydale Hospital Medical Center, Patricia Daehnke for Dr. Andrews, Jennifer M. Renaud for Valleydale Emergency Medical Group, Dr. Harold Morton and William Kent, P.A.

Dr. Andrews earned his undergraduate and medical degrees at Midwestern universities, and did an internship and later a residency in Internal Medicine at Los Angeles County USC Medical Center. In 2000, he began a solo practice in Canoga Park, California in General Internal Medicine. Dr. Andrews was board certified in Internal Medicine.

*****

Of all those deposed, Dr. Andrews was the most difficult to follow and comprehend as he is a man of few words and did not always answer in complete sentences.

*****

Mr. Berger: Doctor, when did you learn that Mr. Folck had been hospitalized in April of 2004?

Dr. Andrews: The day he was admitted.

Mr. Berger: Do you recall how you came to learn of that information, sir?

Dr. Andrews: I believe I got a call from the ER.

Later he said he believed it was a physician who called him. He said that he was told that I went to the ER because of a fever and because I was coughing up blood. Andrews said that he was told that a CT scan showed an infiltrate that identified the problem.

Mr. Berger: Do you recall any questions you may have posed to the Emergency Room physician?

Dr. Andrews: No, I don't.

Mr. Berger: Following receipt of that information, did you attempt to go visit Mr. Folck?

Dr. Andrews: No.

Mr. Berger: During the time Mr. Folck remained hospitalized at that facility did you have any communication with any other healthcare providers, whether it was nurses or doctors, regarding Mr. Folck's condition?

Dr. Andrews said that he had had no contact with either Dr. Morton or Dr. Friedland regarding me or my condition. He also said that he had had no contact with Dr. Soltero, Dr. Amico or Dr. Schwinger about me or my condition.

Dr. Andrews revealed that he had been deposed as a defendant maybe twice in medical negligence cases. One of the cases involved failure to diagnose intestinal lymphoma. The case settled out of court. In the other negligence medical malpractice case he was deposed in, the case was dismissed. He was alleged to have failed to diagnose squamous cell carcinoma.

In the case that settled, Dr. Andrews was put on probation for five years by the Medical Board of California.

Mr. Berger: With respect to the initial interaction with Mr. Folck on March 30, 2004, do you have any recollection of any conversation that may have gone on between you and Ms. LaBelle (office nurse) before you entered the patient's room?

Dr. Andrews: No, I do not.

Dr. Andrews said that he typed his own records and that he performed his own billing. He indicated that he had a telephonic conversation with me on April 10th and that he hand-wrote that entry on my chart the next business day. Raymond Andrews said that I called his voicemail and that he was paged. He said that he had a five-minute phone conversation with me and the gist of my message was that my fever had gone up, again. Continuing, he said that he did not recall if I told him anything else regarding symptoms or complaints. He said that he did not recall me telling him I had night sweats.

*****

As an aside, Dr. Andrews missed the splinter hemorrhages in my fingers, etc. He never looked for them. He seemed single-minded as to what he thought was wrong with me. He said that he did not recall being told I had splinter hemorrhages from the ER doctor who admitted me on April 12th.

*****

Andrews said that after hearing my complaints on April 10th, he told me that I should go to the Emergency Room. His reason being that Andrews saw me on the 9th and I seemed to be getting maybe a little better and then on the 10th the fever was up so I needed a reevaluation.

He told all present that I **refused to go** to the Emergency Room. Andrews said that he did not recall why I told him that I refused to go to the Emergency Room. He said that he thought that I never told him that I presented to the Emergency Room on the three office visits I had with Dr. Andrews.

Andrews admitted that someone from the ER had called him and said that I had been seen at VHMC. He said that he did not remember the date, but that it was before April 12th. He said that he believed that it was an ER physician. Dr. Andrews said he thought that the call was sometime on or after the 6th. He also said that there was **no entry in my chart in his office of that phone call.**

Mr. Berger: Do you have any recollection, sir, as to the gist of the conversation that you had with the Emergency Room physician?

Dr. Andrews: Yes.

Mr. Berger: What was the gist of that conversation?

Dr. Andrews: He had been seen and had a fever. A chest x-ray, I think, was done, and that was negative. I think they did a CBC (complete blood count). His white count was slightly elevated. There was also, I guess, **a blood culture from a previous visit that they thought was a contaminant.**

He added that what he meant by "contaminant" was that an organism grew out of the blood culture. Andrews said that he was not provided with the nature of that organism. He said that he posed no questions to the doctor who called with the information about me. The doctor also said that he never received a copy of the blood contaminant report. He said that he did not ask for a copy of the chest x-ray, nor the CBC.

Mr. Berger: Did you at any time during the office visits that Mr. Folck had on either April 6 or April 9 discuss with him the communication you had received from the Emergency Room physician on or about the 6th of April?

Dr. Andrews: Did we discuss it?

Mr. Berger: Yes, sir.

Dr. Andrews: No.

Mr. Berger: Were you provided with any insight or information from the Emergency Room physician regarding this blood culture contaminant as to what antibiotics should or shouldn't be prescribed to deal with the contaminant?

Dr. Andrews: Not that I recall.

Mr. Berger: How did you know that the antibiotics were potentially dealing with any blood source contaminant that the patient may have had as of April 6?

Dr. Andrews: I wasn't treating a blood source contaminant.

If he wasn't, *who* was?

Andrews said that at no time when he saw me or talked to me on the phone did he attempt to treat a blood source contaminant. Yet, he was told I had one and never dug any further to learn what it was.

Dr. Andrews: I don't think that we're talking about the same thing. When I'm told that the blood culture is positive and that it contains a contaminant, then **the implication is that the organism is not from the blood.** It wasn't in his blood. If I'm told it's a contaminant, to my understanding, that means that it's a skin bacteria picked up during the course when the specimen is drawn.

Yet he never ordered his own culture and sensitivity.

He said that he never reviewed any x-rays (he ordered) of my chest. He relied on the findings of the radiologist.

Dr. Andrews said, regarding antibiotics, that they are not necessarily stronger like Morphine is as compared to Demerol. He said that some antibiotics have broader spectrums of bacteria that they can fight than others do.

Dr. Andrews told all those present that I had described my fever as "intermittent" on the patient intake form for March 30th according to what I told his nurse, Ms. LaBelle.

Mr. Berger: With respect to your medical knowledge and understanding as it existed in March 2004, were there certain patients who were more susceptible to developing sub acute bacterial endocarditis that had risk factors for the development thereof or were predisposed?

Dr. Andrews: I'm not sure. I'd say no.

Mr. Berger: What was the significance, if any, of the patient informing you at the time that his cough had been productive of sputum?

Dr. Andrews: It would tend to indicate that he had an upper respiratory infection.

Mr. Berger: Did the patient describe his sputum any further other than it being dark in nature?

Dr. Andrews: I don't recall anything further.

Dr. Andrews did not think that the dark sputum represented the potential for hemoptysis (bloody sputum). He said that he took between five and ten minutes to perform a limited physical examination of me.

He said that he listened to my heart with his stethoscope as a means to check my cardiovascular system. Andrews said that he did not listen to the carotids. He said that on March 30th, he found nothing unusual and that I had mild bilateral bronchitis.

Dr. Andrews said that on my follow-up visit on April 6th, he did not listen to my heart. He did check my ears, nose, mouth and chest. Raymond Andrews said that my chest revealed mild bilateral bronchitis. He said the bronchitis seemed to be the same that he detected on March 30th.

He said that on April 9th, my temperature was slightly elevated at 100 degrees. He read from his notes on my chart which said, "Patient is in for re-check. He continues to complain of fever though perhaps improved."

Andrews said that his notes indicated my chest x-ray was normal with a slightly elevated white blood count with bilateral bronchitis. He did say that two measures, the alkaline phosphate and the SGOT/SGPT, were both slightly elevated. Andrews said that the three of them taken together indicated a bacterial infection.

Mr. Berger asked whether or not Andrews took any steps after learning that there was a "contaminant" in the blood culture to order a new culture and sensitivity in order to determine whether or not the blood culture was contaminated or not.

Dr. Andrews: No.

Mr. Berger: Were you aware that patients with undiagnosed or untreated bacteria could go on to potentially develop sub acute endocarditis?

Ms. Daehnke: In general?

Mr. Berger: Yes.

Dr. Andrews: Yes.

*****

Like Dr. Morton, Dr. Andrews could have very easily been a hero. He chose to stick to one diagnosis and in my opinion he did not do all he could to learn the nature of my positive blood culture and its resistance to drugs. He answered questions in the deposition like he didn't get it. He seemed to be in his own world with his own set of semantics to follow. His record keeping seemed suspect to me but may have been up to accepted standards.

*****

DEPOSITION OF RON C. FUJITA, MD

Ron C. Fujita, MD was deposed on Monday April 4, 2005 in Northridge, California at the Family Practice Medical Group. The court reporter was Susan Ann Graham. Also present were: Michael Berger, Patricia Daehnke for Dr. Andrews, Robert B. Packer for VHMC, and Nancy L. Flores for Valleydale Emergency Medical Group.

Dr. Fujita earned a B.A. in Biology from a Southern university in 1998. He subsequently received an MD from a Midwestern university college of medicine in 2002. Ron entered the Family Practice Residency Program at Valleydale Hospital in 2002. At the time of his deposition, he was scheduled to graduate in the summer of 2005. Subsequent to that, he went to work as an MD in a Western state.

He stated that as part of his residency he was required to spend clinical hours in the Emergency Room at Valleydale Hospital. Fujita was there for approximately one month, including when he saw me on April 6, 2004 with Harold Morton as his attending physician.

170

Dr. Fujita said that he remembered me as he reviewed my medical records pertaining to April 6th.

Mr. Berger: What do you recall regarding the patient's physical characteristics?

Dr. Fujita: In terms of physical appearance?

Mr. Berger: Yes.

Dr. Fujita: Not really a lot other than he is a Caucasian gentleman who —— this is recorded in the chart, but no acute distress and looks diaphoretic.

Mr. Berger: When you use the term diaphoretic, you are talking about sweating?

Dr. Fujita: Yes.

Dr. Fujita recalled speaking with Dr. Morton approximately three months after seeing me on April 6th. Specifically, Dr. Morton asked about a document known as a face sheet or a T-sheet and why Dr. Morton did not have laboratory reports of me, the patient. Dr. Morton wanted to know about the non-inclusion of the culture and sensitivity results.

Mr. Berger asked Dr. Fujita about speaking with Dr. Andrews over the phone on April 6th. Dr. Fujita said that he spoke with Dr. Andrews at approximately 6:00 pm.

Dr. Fujita: I spoke to Dr. Andrews regarding the previously drawn blood culture (from March 28) that Mr. Folck had.

Mr. Berger: What was the discussion as it relates to the culture and sensitivity report with Dr. Andrews?

Dr. Fujita: As far as I recollect, I told him the information that I have that is documented on the chart that Mr. Folck has blood cultures from March 28th that is positive for *staph aureus* and resistant to penicillin.

Dr. Fujita indicated that Dr. Andrews said he would follow up with me.

Mr. Berger: At any time during the course of this conversation, did Dr. Andrews indicate to you anything along the lines of having the documents that you printed up regarding the culture and sensitivity report faxed to his office for review?

Dr. Fujita: He told me that he would follow up with the patient. I don't know what that specifically entailed. He did not ask me to fax the records over to him specifically.

He further added that Dr. Andrews asked him if I needed to be hospitalized. Fujita said that he thought that I did not require hospitalization.

Dr. Fujita said when he made that statement he was projecting his own opinion and Dr. Morton's opinion.

Dr. Fujita reiterated that he told Dr. Andrews about the *staph* infection and its resistance to penicillin.

Dr. Fujita said that he knew that I was on Augmentin from interviewing me. He said that he knew that Augmentin was a penicillin type antibiotic.

He said that Dr. Andrews told him to continue with the Augmentin.

Dr. Fujita said he did not recollect whether there was any discussion about the possibility of this blood culture being a "contaminant" or if he stated that to Dr. Andrews. He said that he told Dr. Andrews that the x-ray results looked normal.

Dr. Fujita said that from the lab results, etc., in addition to the bacterial infection, that I might have a viral infection and possibly a stress reaction which elevated my white blood count.

Mr. Berger asked if Dr. Fujita examined my fingers when he gave me a physical examination on April 6th.

Dr. Fujita said he had no recollection of splinter hemorrhages.

Fujita said that he did not hear any murmurs, gallops or any abnormal sounds when he listened to my heart and that if he had heard anything he would have noted it on the chart.

Dr. Fujita said that he knew that I presented the symptom of an intermittent fever that had gone on for nine days.

Fujita said that he did not recollect Dr. Morton express to him any concern that Augmentin might not be the right antibiotic for me.

*****

Ron C. Fujita, MD also had an opportunity to be a hero on April 6th. However, he, too, missed clues that were available and ignored the obvious wrong choice of Augmentin to treat my *Staphylococcus aureus* infection. Like Dr. Morton and Dr. Andrews, he had his own interpretation of what was going on with me. I was, in effect, his practice test dummy for concurring with an improper antibiotic for what ailed me.

*****

Someone very close to me had a few choice words to say about Dr. Morton, Dr. Andrews and Dr. Fujita or, as she called them, "The Three Stooges."

She said, "They all sound like a bunch of bumbling idiots. I find it amazing that the news is run every hour and they repeat the same stuff which has like little or no importance. You know, like which of the Kardashian sisters has the biggest butt? And yet the stories go on, untold, swept aside quietly, settled for a dollar amount that will never replace what had been lost. But the person who caused the suffering isn't even affected by it because they have insurance for it, and have their practice covered by limited liability. So, you can never really hit them where it hurts."

She also told me that she wanted the three doctors injected with the same bacterium I had so that they could endure what I had endured to see how they liked it.

173

The three doctors in question were caught up in their own worlds with blinders on and no collective or individual common sense while 'the elephant' came charging at me. They offered excuses for their actions. I say to each of them, "Your excuse is so lame that it ought to be on crutches!"

THE "SLAP AND TICKLE" INCIDENT

Sometime in April 2005, I received a phone call from Lobl's office that VHMC and Dr. Morton, through their respective attorneys, wanted to have a "voluntary" settlement conference in Century City.

I cannot recall the name of the firm that offered the services. For all I knew, it could have been "Screw the Injured Party for a Fee Settlement Services."

I drove to one of the large, tall office buildings in Century City.

I snaked my way around in an underground parking garage on several levels. Finally, I found a spot and recorded it on the parking ticket and made my way to an elevator.

I was in a so-so mood as I arrived at the offices where I had been directed. At least there had been some movement in the case. I was curious to see what was afoot but cautious and skeptical about what I might learn.

*****

Once inside, I was met by Michael Berger. Rick Lobl was not there as he had other legal business to attend to.

As we went toward a small office, I saw the defendant attorneys and other people all sitting around a large conference table in a room with lots of windows.

The idea of the meeting was to start a dialogue and, hopefully for the defendants, negotiate an out-of-court settlement that was favorable for them and not me.

The lead person for the settlement service was a retired judge from the Santa Monica Superior Court who was earning a fee to represent the defendants. That's right; he was a silver-haired, silver-tongued devil who was called a "mediator."

The Judge was hoping to settle the case on terms favorable to the defendant insurance companies so that they might employ him in the future to clean some other plaintiffs' clocks monetarily.

I listened to what the old judge had to say. I surmised that he had barely glanced at the merits of the case and had not bothered himself with many of the significant details. Never mind what was involved. The Judge only wanted another notch in his "settlement gun." I picked up on that right away.

Michael Berger did bring up salient points about our side of the case. However, his effort was nothing to write home about.

I was hearing all kinds of b.s. from the Judge about the plaintiffs' positions, and I let him know in no uncertain terms that I was highly pissed off at what had happened to me. I said that I would have future medical costs, including at least one open-heart surgery in the future to replace the human tissue valve now in my chest.

The Judge left the room and went into "The Den of Thieves." (I considered the room with all the defense people in it to be "The Den of Thieves.")

*****

A long time later, the Judge returned, and after a lot of meaningless talk from him, he informed Michael Berger and me that the two defendants, collectively, would pay 50% of $300,000 to settle their cases with me. In other words, they collectively wanted to buy me off for a total of $150,000 in some sort of split-fee arrangement.

My blood pressure went sky high. My nostrils flared. I got a very angry look on my face as I glared at the Judge.

"The surgery I just went through cost $250,000. I have all the bills. And that says nothing about the pain and suffering."

The Judge said, "The defendants calculated that a future open-heart surgery will cost $35,000."

I said, "Will they be getting that from a Cracker Jack box or will that be a Third World surgery?! That is crap."

The Judge said, "Give me something I can work with."

I said, "Why would I do that?"

He said, "The defendants say that you couldn't have been that sick since you drove yourself to the Emergency Room on April 12th, 2004."

"Not sick?! I was dying. Apparently you did not read the medical records!"

The Judge said, "Once you got the infection, the surgery was inevitable and nothing could have prevented it."

I said, "The only thing that prevented me from dying was me and not those jack offs. By the way, your honor, have you ever had your aortic valve in a vegetative state and had triple pneumonia due to gross negligence medical malpractice?"

He did not respond.

I said, "If what you said was true, then there would be no need for drugs like Levaquin if all cases of bacterial endocarditis from *Staphylococcus Aureus* resulted in surgery."

He sat there silent. Mr. Berger said nothing as I glared at the Judge.

"The fact of the matter is that most cases of bacterial endocarditis are resolved without surgery. The statistics are clear about that."

The Judge said that the fact of the matter was that these sorts of cases settled for $290,000.

I said, in a raised voice, "*You* do not have any of my interests in settling this case. You are a hired gun by the defense. You can say whatever you want but you have no authority, legally, to make me settle — none!"

The thieves in the conference room were lying through their teeth at all costs to save their clients' money. This distasteful exchange between plaintiff and defendants was allowed since there was no law against it. They could lie through their collective teeth and smack me around and it was not illegal.

*****

As I saw it, the lawyers were hiding behind the "Hypocritical Oath" they took when they became lawyers. What I mean is that a lawyer, by law, not by morals, can step outside himself in the name of the law, if he chooses to, and beat down an opposing party by any means to achieve a better outcome for his client. Including lying. Lawyers have a "right" to "defend" their clients under the law. If someone thinks that a lawyer is lying, it has to be proven in court. They are not sworn in court to tell the truth. It is supposed to be that they are truthful being officers of the court. However, I don't think that that has any bearing on the yarns some of them spin on behalf of their clients.

It sickens me to think that the truth will be stretched or lies will be told in medical malpractice cases. I think that it happens all the time and that some lawyers are part of this playing with the truth.

I seriously doubt if many medical malpractice defense attorneys would let a family member or close friend go through what some plaintiffs endure in a medical malpractice case. Yet they heap it on plaintiffs.

I'm speaking about some medical malpractice defense attorneys, not all.

To me, it's all hypocrisy under the guise of being a lawyer.

*****

Getting back to the old judge, I told him, "There is a possibility that I may need two future open-heart surgeries since no one can say with any certainty how long replacement valves really last. My asking price is $750,000. I don't give a damn what you think the value of my case is since you are not a medical expert nor a medical economist and you don't know squat about my case! You didn't even have your facts straight!"

Then I turned to Mr. Berger and got into it with him. I said, "I am aghast that Lobl has not employed a medical cost economist to prepare a valuation of my case prior to this meeting and, furthermore, I seem to be the only one in the room standing up for me! Also, not all of the people who should be named as defendants in this case have been named. And I mean Dr. Andrews. Should I give you guys the boot and say it's me against the world?!"

I waited for a response and none was forthcoming. Then I said, "I'm outta here!"

I continued to bellow as I walked out. It was an incredible waste of three hours of my time!

*****

When I got to a large window at the front of the conference room, I stopped and glared at "The Thieves." Each of them saw how upset I was.

Just before I headed for the main door, I flipped them off with both hands.

I passed Linda Rurangirwa (Dr. Andrews' attorney) on my way out and she asked, "How did it go?"

I said, "It went like s—t!"

She had not been privy to the discussions in the conference room since Dr. Andrews was not named as a plaintiff on the lawsuit.

I was so mad that I did $2,000 damage to my Toyota Tundra truck as I exited the parking structure. I caved in one side of the bed of my truck leaving and scraped one corner of my front bumper by hitting a concrete structure.

I drove home but I was irate.

*****

As soon as I walked in the door, I called Lobl's office and yelled at Michael Berger in a profanity-laced tirade up one side and down the other over what had happened at the "settlement conference."

I told Berger that I was not flying blind in the case, that I had an attorney on the defense side of medical malpractice cases that I was consulting with. Additionally, I told Berger that they were blowing the case and that they were lazy!

It had just been another day at the office for the defense attorneys and their experts — no big deal to them.

I finished my lambasting of Mr. Berger and hung up.

*****

A little while later, Rick Lobl called and I gave it to him. Then he told me that there would be no further tirades on my part to anyone from his office. Rick said that I was not to talk like that to anyone in his office who was involved in the case or they would drop their representation of me. He also said that he didn't want me to talk to any other attorney about the case.

A little later I said to him, "You need to get it in gear, Rick. So far you haven't done that much and I'm not going to go away for a quick and dirty settlement. Got it?"

The next day, I called my first ex-wife, Wendy Redfield, again, and told her what had transpired. She was not shocked and asked me who the attorneys were and the law firms. My ex said that she knew them and that this was the way they responded all the time.

I had given Wendy a lot of information about my case and she characterized it as a "slam dunk loser" case for the defendants.

Talking to herself, Wendy said, "Can we get this guy half a million dollars for his injuries?" She was saying this about my situation indicating what all the lawyers on both sides of my case should agree to as far as a settlement.

She said that if either the hospital or Dr. Morton had been her clients, she would have told them to settle and get it off the judicial calendar.

They were attempting to do that, but for pennies.

She told me, "You do not want to take a case like this to court if you're a defendant. The liability is crystal clear, no matter what the defendants might say."

GIVE 'TIL IT HURTS

In early May 2004, I received a letter in the mail from Valleydale Hospital Medical Center.

The first part of the letter told a tale about a store owner in the San Fernando Valley who was shot with a handgun during a robbery attempt. The bullet went all the way through the right ventricle of his heart eventually lodging in his back. Quick-thinking bystanders immediately called 911 and an emergency unit responded. That unit was directed to take the critically wounded man to Valleydale Hospital Medical Center.

The fast-acting doctors, nurses and other hospital personnel got the man to surgery eleven minutes after arriving at the hospital. The man lived through the emergency surgery and 56 days later, he went home to resume his life.

The letter told me that the hospital thought that every patient needing emergency care should receive prompt and proper attention even if they did not have a life-threatening gunshot wound. The letter assured me that the doctors and other personnel in the emergency room and trauma center always gave patients 100% effort no matter what ailed the patient.

The last part of the letter asked me for a financial contribution to help the emergency room and trauma center purchase technologically advanced equipment to improve patient care.

The letter was signed by Stephen E. Jones who was the Medical Director of Emergency Services.

*****

I want you to think about what it might have been like for each and every one of you to have been in my shoes reading that letter given what had happened to me at the Valleydale Hospital ER. Please give yourself a couple of minutes to do that before you continue reading.

I closed my eyes as I slowly and carefully set down the letter so as not to destroy it. Then it hit me.

I thought to myself, "Those idiot bastards. How dare they have the gall to send me this letter?"

After I went into my backyard, I went ICBM (inter-continental ballistic missile) on anything and everything in sight of me. I broke a couple wooden chairs, smashed clay flower pots, jumped on two metal folding chairs and flattened them, and ripped out two clothesline poles set in concrete using only my feet to kick them and my hands to pull them out.

About fifteen minutes later, still huffing and puffing, I sat down on my couch and bawled my eyes out. Once the crying stopped, I called Shelley and told her about the letter.

Shelley was incensed. She thought it was unbelievably cruel to get a letter asking for a donation to the Valleydale ER when they had totally screwed up my *Staphylococcus aureus* infection. Shelley had totally gotten it about the donation letter.

I finished my call, typed a letter to Rick Lobl, photocopied the hospital letter and delivered them both to his office.

Lobl called back and downplayed the whole thing. He said it was just a form letter that had been sent out since I had been a former patient.

*****

A month later, I got a second letter from VHMC asking for a donation to the ER fund.

This time I fired off a letter to the hospital CEO telling him who I was, what I had endured at the hands of his hospital ER and hospital personnel, and what I thought about their donation letter.

Soon, some days later, I received a letter saying that I had been removed from the hospital mailing list.

Then Rick Lobl called. "I told you that I don't want you talking to the defense! You shouldn't have written that letter to them!"

I shot back, "You didn't do a thing about stopping those letters so I did! And if I get any more letters from them about donations to the ER—"

Interrupting me in mid-sentence, he said, "If you contact the defense again, I am dropping you as a client. Don't do it. I'm sorry that you got the letters, but they were form letters and we have a case against them. Let it go."

I wanted to tell Lobl to stick it but I didn't. Rick was at his best as a persuasive, manipulative attorney at that moment.

My feeling was that there was some sort of a game going on.

I backed off. Yet to this day I am miffed about why he didn't contact them to stop the letters, even when I had asked him to. I guess he had his "closed club" to think about. Apparently that meant that his client should bear the brunt of things like the letters without him intervening. It would all become clear to me at a later date as to why he acted the way that he did.

DEPOSITION OF BINA SEHMI

It was finally necessary to get a few details from Bina Sehmi about attempts to contact me with the news of my blood infection.

On Monday June 13, 2005, Bina Sehmi was deposed at Valleydale Hospital Medical Center. Joseph R. Lombardi was the court reporter. Those present included: Michael Berger, Sara Clark for Valleydale Hospital Medical Center, Linda Rurangirwa for Dr. Andrews, Richard Ryan for Valleydale Emergency Medical Group and Harold Morton, MD.

Bina Sehmi, a ward clerk in the Emergency Room at VHMC for six and a half years, said that she never interacted with me at the hospital nor had any face-to-face conversations with me there. She also said that she never spoke to me on the phone.

Mr. Berger asked Bina if she was aware of or had knowledge of a document titled "Subject Recall Notification of Results" published by VHMC.

When Mr. Berger showed it to her, she stated that she had never seen it before then.

Bina stated that on numerous occasions she had been asked to contact patients at the request of the ER doctors. However, she did not give the results of any lab work. She said that she never gave results.

Ms. Sehmi said that she contacted patients by phone and then let the doctor who requested the call talk to the patient.

Bina said that she had tried to contact me at the request of Dr. Morton so that Dr. Morton could talk to me. Specifically, Morton told Bina that he wanted to discuss the results of a positive blood culture with me.

Bina said she got a face sheet with my information on it, including my phone numbers. She said that there was a work number listed and a home phone number.

Ms. Sehmi said that she tried to call me four times before her shift ended at 7:00 pm on the day Dr. Morton spoke with her. She said that she tried to call me at home.

On the first attempt, Bina dialed a wrong number. Someone answered the phone and said that I didn't live there. So, she called the work number and no one picked up. Later, on the second attempt to contact me at my home phone number, she got the same wrong number that she did on the first attempt.

She called the number again and got the same wrong number. At that point, she told Morton that she had not been able to contact me.

Bina said that she was never requested to send a certified letter or certified mail to a patient who she had been unable to contact by phone. She said that Dr. Morton did not ask her to send a certified letter or any certified mail to me requesting me to contact the Emergency Department. Ms. Sehmi said that she had never had to do that.

Mr. Berger: At some point on the same day that was requested of you by Dr. Morton to contact Mr. Folck, did you have occasion to see Dr. Friedland in the Emergency Department?

Ms. Sehmi: Yes.

Mr. Berger: Did you have any conversation with Dr. Friedland regarding a patient by the name of David Folck at that time?

Ms. Sehmi: I did not.

She said that she heard a conversation between Morton and Friedland. She added that Morton told Friedland of the culture and sensitivity results of the blood culture, and that Morton also said that they had been unable to reach me by phone. At that point, she said, Friedland called his office to get my home phone information.

Bina said that she did not hear Morton identify the organism found. She said that a person at Dr. Friedland's office gave her the same phone numbers for me that VHMC had for me.

According to her, Friedland called his office and asked his office person to give Bina the numbers.

Bina recalled listening to Dr. Morton. She recalled that Morton said, "Look, I can't get a hold of this guy. Nobody knows him at these numbers."

She also stated that it was her understanding that she was not to proceed with further contact attempts to reach me that day.

Bina said that she had a later conversation with Dr. Morton about trying to contact me.

Ms. Sehmi: Dr. Morton was passing me by. I was standing outside, and he did stop by and say, "Hey, do you remember that guy, David Folck?" And he had to kind of jog my memory. And I said, "Oh, the guy we tried to call?" And he said, "Yes." He said, "Well, they're suing me." And I said, "Oh, I'm sorry to hear that." And he said—I said, "But we tried really hard to get a hold of him. We tried the numbers. We didn't get through. What were we supposed to do, Dr. Morton?" He said, at that point, "I suppose that we should have sent a letter."

She said that she was the person who notified Dr. Morton of my blood culture results. Bina spoke to him as she showed him the culture results.

Ms. Sehmi: This is your patient. Do you remember?

She said that Morton asked, "Can you try to get him on the phone for me?"

Bina said that the culture and the sensitivity are reported on two different documents. First comes the culture, and the sensitivity follows maybe two days later on the system in use at VHMC on the day when she tried to call me. She said that lab results automatically generate a printout no matter if they are positive or not.

186

Bina reiterated that she made notes on the face sheet but not on the actual patient chart since she only had the face sheet and not my chart regarding her phone attempts.

Mr. Berger: The person that spoke with you in your attempts to contact Mr. Folck's residence on those three occasions, did that person — respond to you in Spanish or English?

Ms. Sehmi: It was accented English.

Mr. Berger: Did you ever attempt to contact the operator to see if the lines had been crossed or any other potential as far as your inability to get a hold of the patient?

Ms. Sehmi: I'm sorry. No.

She said that she was not aware of any other attempts by any other person to contact me.

DEPOSITION OF L. JEROME ROBERT FRIEDLAND, MD

Dr. Friedland was deposed on Tuesday June 14, 2005 at the Orthopedic Medical Center in Reseda, California. Victoria L. Valine was the court reporter. Those in attendance included: Michael Berger, Sara Clark for VHMC, Michael D. Attar for Harold Morton and the Valleydale Emergency Medical Group, Patricia Daehnke for Dr. Andrews, and Linda Star for Dr. Friedland.

Doctor Friedland had been a practicing orthopedic surgeon for more than thirty years when he was deposed. He stated that he had given one hundred depositions and that five of them had to do with his opinion as an expert witness. Friedland had been the treating physician in 80% of the cases.

In general, Dr. Friedland did not recall or remember interactions with Bina Sehmi or Dr. Morton or Dr. Andrews relating to my infection problem and did not recall or remember ordering me to go to VHMC to have my knee tapped and drained on March 28, 2004.

When asked if he thought over the years he treated me (1999 to present) that I had been a compliant patient, he said that I had been very compliant.

Dr. Friedland said that it would not be within the scope of his practice to order a blood culture and sensitivity. Dr. Friedland said that an orthopedic specialist would only order a blood culture if he were evaluating a patient.

He did say that there were times when he sent a patient to the ER at Valleydale and told the physician on duty, for example, to look at a patient's knee and that, if it looked swollen, to tap it and do a fluid culture. Friedland said that the only recollections of my visits to him for March and April of 2004 were from his office notes in the patient record. He did indicate that I mentioned to him while an arthroscopic procedure on my right knee was being considered that I had a respiratory problem and that he told me that it might have to be postponed.

*****

"The Experts" for both sides were up next and they had plenty of interesting things to say about the case.

Chapter 13—The Experts

The question on the table was this: Who were the "real" experts evaluating my case and who were the "faux" experts?

The second question at hand was: Which experts would be **more believable?**

*****

Even though my dissatisfaction with Rick Lobl was growing, I continued to retain his firm. I also continued to talk with my first ex-wife Wendy about what was going on.

Lobl seemed to be pursuing a strategy of getting something for almost nothing. He and Michael Berger deposed everyone associated with the mishandling of my infection, but there wasn't much movement after that.

I told Lobl that he should prepare for a trial because I was not satisfied with the offers from the two defendants — VHMC and Dr. Morton. He gave me the once-over as I sat in his office after I told him this, like he didn't really believe that it was what I wanted.

Lobl reminded me, "You know that they want to settle."

"I get that. I won't do it for pennies on the dollar and that's what they are proposing. Screw them."

"You don't go to trial against a defendant who wants to settle out of court. I sense that you want to grind them up, that you are angry with them and you want to slam them in court."

"I don't care about them!"

"They have the purse strings. They won't take kindly to you trying to flame them in public. They will make it unpleasant for you. They are going to say things that you won't like."

"Do we have a good case or not?"

"We do and we don't."

"That's *not* what you've been telling me until now!"

"You have to be objective about this sort of thing. There is a downside to these cases if they go to trial. Juries are a wild card. This case has a lot of technical medical stuff involved. A jury might turn a deaf ear to it."

"That's why I hired you."

We went back and forth for a while longer and then I told him that I was sticking to my guns. He said, "Ok."

At this point, no money had changed hands between Lobl and I and none had been asked for.

His was a "boutique" law firm, not one with numerous attorneys. He and Michael Berger were THE attorneys — period.

*****

I emailed my first ex-wife Wendy and asked her if she had any take on who might be good experts for a case like mine. She suggested several people. One of the medical experts Wendy mentioned was Robert L. Shuman, MD.

She wrote:

"Robert L. Shuman, MD. Cardiothoracic surgeon. 562-XXX-XXXX. In Long Beach, California. He usually does defense work. He doesn't like Rick Lobl so he may not help you but he is a very good expert, so I would try.

Other stuff: Keep in mind that if you have not settled by the fiftieth day prior to the trial date, you will need to designate experts and so will the defense by law."

She told me that the experts also needed to be deposed as part of the discovery process.

Wendy estimated that the costs of the experts could get into tens of thousands of dollars.

She also mentioned:

"Also discuss with Michael Berger or Rick their thoughts on serving defendants with a CCP (California Code of Civil Procedure) 998 offer. It is a statutory offer to settle your case for a specific amount.

For example, you could serve a 998 offer on the ER doctor for $500,000. He has thirty days to accept the offer. If he doesn't accept and the case goes to trial and if you recover a verdict in excess of the $500,000, then he will have to pay your trial costs including your experts' fees. An offer can be made to each of the defendants individually and that is the best way. You can get some small change from a defendant that you don't think has much liability to help fund your case against the other defendants or also to knock off a part of the apportionment issues between defendants and maximize recovery from the target. Another strategy would be to keep all defendants in the case and have them point the finger at each other. If that happens, you will win. Good luck."

Rick Lobl never even mentioned any of the above to me. Lobl went about garnering experts. So did the defendants. I waited.

*****

Sometime later, once the experts had been designated and depositions began, I had to go back into Lobl's office to sign something. So I did.

While I sat there, I saw a stack of photocopied documents. It turned out that they were from one Ray Brinkman, MD. Lobl had contacted Dr. Brinkman to get the latest in the medical literature about cases similar to mine. Later, we learned that Brinkman had been hired as a defense witness by the other side.

I asked Rick Lobl, "What are those?"

Lobl seemed none too happy to have to wade through the stack of documents.

He mentioned, "They are from Dr. Brinkman. When I first started as a medical malpractice attorney, I worked on the defense side. We retained Dr. Brinkman as one of our experts. The case involved a plastic surgeon who had really screwed up someone, her face I believe."

Lobl seemed tired of me and my case. At least that is what I sensed.

In that previous case, Lobl knew that the plastic surgeon was liable for malpractice. However, he was not sure if there were mitigating circumstances that might lessen the financial settlement. He called upon Dr. Brinkman for help.

On his first and only meeting with Dr. Brinkman on that case he asked Dr. Brinkman what he thought. Lobl said that the doctor in not so many words indicated he was open to suggestions from Lobl about what he might say.

Rick dropped him like a hot potato and settled the case out of court.

As I write this, I find it ironic that at that time Rick Lobl wanted me to believe Rick was altogether ethical. I'll explain later.

*****

DEPOSITION OF RAY BRINKMAN, MD

Dr. Brinkman was deposed on July 19, 2005. Martin Spee was the court reporter. Michael Berger represented me. Patricia Daehnke represented Dr. Andrews. Jennifer Renaud represented Valleydale Emergency Medical Group and Dr. Morton.

Ray Brinkman said that he had been deposed over 200 times in twenty-five years. He said that he reviewed records from VHMC, Dr. Soltero, Dr. Friedland, Dr. Amico, Dr. Andrews and another volume from Dr. Friedland.

He said that he also reviewed the depositions of everyone in the case, except Dr. Friedland's deposition.

Brinkman added that he reviewed x-rays of mine from September 10, 2002, February 18, 2003, and June 21, 2004; a CT scan of my chest dated April 12, 2004; a nuclear cardiology study from April 16, 2004; and a series of x-rays of my chest from April 2, April 6, April 12, April 19, April 21, April 22, and April 25 — all from 2004).

He also reviewed several taped echocardiograms of my chest and heart.

Ray Brinkman reviewed medical literature as well.

He said that he planned to make some demonstrative drawings for trial to explain his take on what had happened.

Dr. Brinkman was then asked by Michael Berger if any of the cases where he was retained as an expert involved endocarditis or *Staphylococcus aureus* endocarditis.

The doctor replied that it was a common topic that came up both in his own practice and as an expert. He didn't know how many cases of endocarditis he had reviewed over the years.

Dr. Brinkman said that he had about five cases of endocarditis currently under review in different states.

He stated that he practiced both cardiology as well as internal medicine.

Dr. Brinkman acknowledged that I had *Staphylococcus aureus* on my aortic heart valve. He said that he had seen twenty-five cases of a similar nature.

Continuing, he said that virtually every one of them had gone on to have the aortic valve replaced. Brinkman said that he could not remember any one of them who did not have replacement valve surgery, even if they did not need it when he first saw them. He said that some of them delayed the surgery for a year or two. But that everyone who got *Staphylococcus aureus* endocarditis ended up with surgery.

That was the gist of Dr. Brinkman's opinion. He believed that no matter who did or didn't do what, where, when or why, I would have required

193

my aortic valve to be replaced once my heart valve was infected. Brinkman offered up that the new valve I received would last in the neighborhood of twenty years with the technique and valve Dr. Soltero used.

He said that he would not be providing an opinion as to the standard of care I received. Dr. Brinkman was only used to offer causation and damages.

Under questioning, Dr. Brinkman said that I had pre-existing abnormalities on my aortic valve that predisposed me to this infection which was an additional risk factor for this valve replacement at some time. In other words, with or without this infection, a heart valve replacement would have been necessary in the future due to abnormalities. He said that given my life expectancy that I would not require a future aortic valve replacement.

He said that I would require future medical visits and/or medications and tests and related procedures for the rest of my life.

Dr. Brinkman said that in my older x-rays I had mild **cardiomegaly** or heart chamber enlargement. He said that this indicated a prior heart valve condition.

What he meant was that my heart chamber enlarged since my heart valve, in his opinion, was not fully functioning. This caused more blood in the heart chamber than should have been there with a healthy valve and hence an expansion of the chamber over time. **Dr. Brinkman felt that this had gone on for four years or more.**

Ray Brinkman said that he saw no notation in my records that I had been treated for cardiomegaly in the past; that is, it had never been mentioned.

He also said he could tell there were other heart problems with my heart as evidenced by the increased thickness of the left ventricle. Brinkman ruled out everything but aortic valve disease as the cause. He said that I might not have known it because it might not create symptoms for years.

Ray Brinkman had no idea of the origin of the infection.

In the doctor's opinion, a murmur may or may not have been there before the infection and it might have been there but may not have been loud enough to hear.

He said that I likely had the infection there for weeks. Dr. Brinkman said that the infection probably started in my knee and went to my heart and that the vegetative growth was quite large upon discovery, indicating that it had been there for some time.

Brinkman said that a person could get *Staphylococcus aureus* in his bloodstream, and he might or might not get endocarditis. He said it could infect a valve or not. The doctor felt that the whole scenario was highly variable.

The doctor indicated that with all endocarditis, the patient will be better with medication and surgery together and especially with *Staphylococcus aureus* endocarditis, the kind that I had.

Dr. Brinkman said that in order to have avoided the need for surgery, the treatment of the *Staphylococcus aureus* in my body needed to have started **as of March 30, 2004**.

He said that generally he thought there was a delay between the time of endocarditis and the time a patient gets in to see the doctor.

Regarding the vegetation on my heart as shown on the first taped echocardiogram, he said it looked friable — like it might break off — which is typical of *Staphylococcus aureus* on a heart valve. He said that the surgery corrected the enlarged chambers due to cardiac insufficiency.

*****

This was a confusion defense at work with Ray Brinkman being the point man.

The defense was set to argue that I had pre-existing heart conditions prior to the infection, even though there was **not one shred of evidence** from any cardiologist or taped echocardiogram to back that up. Dr. Brinkman only used some previous x-rays, which are not the prevailing standard of care for such a diagnosis.

Never mind that I was a big guy and that, as a result, my heart chamber might have been bigger than heart chambers smaller men might have in their hearts.

Dr. Brinkman offered no precise measurements as to what constituted cardiomegaly in my body, meaning how large was "enlarged" as far as my heart chamber. Opinions without backup facts are not a good idea to set forth during a trial.

I called my first ex-wife Wendy and told her that Ray Brinkman had given a deposition in my case for the defense.

She said, "Oh, God — they're desperate. He does not have a good reputation for either side. Most medical malpractice attorneys know that if the other side uses him, they are desperate."

*****

Would my side have an expert who could shed more objective light on this argument?

DEPOSITION OF ROBERT L. SHUMAN, MD

Robert L. Shuman, MD, was deposed on Thursday July 28, 2005 at his office in Long Beach, California. The court reporter was Lucia Moskal. Michael Berger was there on my behalf. Richard Ryan represented Valleydale Emergency Medical Group and Dr. Morton. Sara Clark represented Valleydale Hospital Medical Center. Linda K. Rurangirwa represented Dr. Andrews.

Dr. Shuman was a well-known and highly regarded cardiac surgeon, thoracic surgeon and major peripheral vascular surgeon. He had a sterling reputation among medical malpractice attorneys on both sides.

Shuman was designated an expert witness on my side. He had worked a lot of cases on the defense side of medical malpractice, but when he heard the circumstances of my case from Rick Lobl he agreed to be a plaintiff's expert.

Shuman graduated from Wake Forest University in 1966 then from the Bowman Gray School of Medicine in Winston-Salem, North Carolina in 1970. After that, he interned at the University of Chicago Hospital and Clinics in 1970 and 1971. He completed a General Surgery Residency at UCSD Hospital in San Diego in 1976. In 1979, he completed a Cardiovascular Thoracic Surgery Residency at Rush Presbyterian St. Luke's Medical Center. By all accounts, he was a surgeon's surgeon in his areas of specialty.

He stated that in his career, he had given well over 200 depositions and had testified at trial over one hundred times. This was over the course of twenty-three years.

The doctor shared that he had been retained as an expert over 600 times in twenty-three years.

He said that over the years he had testified for the defense about 75% of the time.

Shuman said that he had only given a deposition in one case involving endocarditis and an aortic valve replacement.

As an aside, I told my first ex-wife Wendy that Dr. Shuman was to be an expert witness for my side. She was ecstatic at the news. She said, simply, "He is the best for heart cases."

Mr. Ryan: In cardiothoracic surgery parlance, what does a successful surgery mean?

Dr. Shuman: Well, he operated on the patient for the proper indication. He had a successful operation in that the patient lived, the valve was placed well, the homograft (human tissue valve), and he is doing relatively well now from the standpoint of his valve. I understand that he's not been able to go back to work.

Mr. Ryan: Have you formed any opinion as to why he can't go back to work?

Dr. Shuman: Not completely, no.

Mr. Ryan: When you say "not completely," it sounds like you may have a partial opinion.

Dr. Shuman: Well, I know that he has orthopedic problems, I know that he has depression, and he has the cardiac event. So all of those are together, and I wasn't clear when I read his deposition exactly — I know that he is not looking for work at this time, but I don't think that that precluded him from going back to work at some time.

He said that 75% of those who are capable of working or who were working prior to heart valve surgery, in his experience, return to work after the surgery.

Dr. Shuman said that he would not be testifying to the standard of care I received from any defendant.

Mr. Ryan: In the context of this type of valve replacement surgery, what is an excellent result?

Dr. Shuman: Well, it's a complex valve replacement. You want to be able to replace the aortic valve, and try and eliminate all of the infection and prevent further abscess formation, and Dr. Soltero was able to do that. Basically, it's to restore the competency of the aortic valve. The eradication of the organism, you're only doing that by debridement, but you're relying on the antibiotics to do that primarily. So you debride as much tissue as necessary to eliminate any that might be infected, although you know that you're obviously going to leave some behind, and you have to rely on the antibiotics to do that. So surgery is never truly meant to eradicate the infection. It's meant to restore the competency of the aortic valve. It's meant to eliminate the vegetation, which was quite large and had a propensity to break off and produce a stroke. So, all of those goals were met.

He said the remaining organism is eradicated with antibiotics by diffusion.

Mr. Ryan: Do I also understand correctly that it is difficult by antibiotics alone to eradicate large vegetation?

Mr. Berger: Let me just object. It's an incomplete hypothetical. You're not providing the doctor with any determination as to when the vegetation occurred, how long the growth was present.

Mr. Ryan: How large was the vegetation here?

Dr. Shuman: They described it as "greater than 10 mm."

Dr. Shuman said that it meant, to him, 10-12 mms in size.

Mr. Ryan: Is it true that by replacing this valve, that the heart actually — the atrium and ventricle actually became healthier afterwards?

Mr. Berger: Objection. It's vague and ambiguous as to the term "healthier."

Dr. Shuman: They would become smaller, not dilated.

Mr. Ryan: Which is healthier; correct?

Dr. Shuman: Yes.

Dr. Shuman indicated that the two had been dilated as seen on the two taped echocardiograms. He agreed that Dr. Schwinger had said that the degree of dilation was "quite severely dilated."

Dr. Shuman: Well, all of this (dilation) was due to the fact that the aortic valve was leaking. When you have a situation where the aortic valve suddenly starts leaking, the ventricle has to respond, and it responds by stretching and dilating. As it stretches and dilates, it's going to allow the left atrium to stretch and dilate as well, and that is associated with acute aortic insufficiency, which is related to endocarditis. Once you restore the aortic valve to a competent valve, you no longer have that overload on the left ventricle. So, it accepts the blood, it ejects it, it doesn't fall back into the ventricle. So, in time, as you repeat echocardiograms, that ventricle and atrium will get smaller.

Shuman said that the cause of the stretching was blood volume overload from acute aortic regurgitation.

Mr. Ryan: Do you have an opinion as to whether or not there is a sufficient body of literature (for U.S. patients) describing the longevity of homografts used in this type of case?

Dr. Shuman: The literature is what we would call mid-term. In other words, the longevity to follow these patients, you like to have ten-year follow-up. There are isolated reports. Most of the follow-up of significant numbers

199

would be termed five-year mid-term follow-up. But **the problems that are occurring are that the homografts are not lasting anywhere near as long as they had hoped** that they would. So the durability of the homograft is a very major concern.

Mr. Ryan: I understand that the expectation is that these homografts will last at least ten to fifteen years. Is that incorrect?

Dr. Shuman: That was the original expectation. That has proved not to be true over time.

Mr. Ryan: Was a homograft a good choice for Mr. Folck?

Dr. Shuman: I think it was.

Mr. Wright: Why is that?

Dr. Shuman: Well, there is a slight, a tiny, slight difference in the ability to infect a homograft versus a mechanical valve. But it's very, very slight, and so Dr. Soltero was going to try to do the homograft. If he was not able to do that, he was going to insert a St. Jude (mechanical) valve, which would have been fine.

Shuman said that he did not do homografts in his practice. He said that they were not lasting as long as expected due to calcification.

Robert Shuman said that his expectation was that I could end up with a mechanical valve when a replacement valve was needed and that there would be a more involved surgery than the first time around with an entire aortic root replacement necessary and bypasses of the coronary arteries as well. He said more than one replacement surgery was possibly necessary in my case. Shuman said that when you do a replacement surgery, you tell a patient ten years.

Mr. Ryan: You would agree that Mr. Folck's hospitalization here was a complicated hospitalization, and that a revision surgery would be less complicated in terms of the overall complications that were treated here and the length of the stay, et cetera?

Dr. Shuman: I wouldn't agree with that at all. This was a very straightforward situation. I wouldn't call his hospitalization complicated from the standpoint that he came in, he had antibiotics, and he went to surgery. He really had no post-operative complication, and was able to be discharged quickly.

Mr. Ryan: What I meant to say, this was lengthier than a revision surgery would be.

Dr. Shuman: Correct.

Mr. Ryan: So there were other procedures and therapies rendered here that wouldn't be rendered in a future revision surgery; correct?

Mr. Berger: Well, let me just object. I think that probably calls for speculation, is an incomplete hypothetical.

Dr. Shuman: Well, he was in the hospital for eleven days, and on a revision surgery, if you assume that everything is done as an outpatient, the TEE and the heart catheter, you're then going to come in and have the heart surgery. Even if you're at nine days, that's assuming no complications whatsoever. As you're doing a revision, you're going to be very close to the conduction system, so there is a possible need for a pacemaker. Often what you do is you look at a very slow heart rate. You hope the edema will subside. That means that they have to stay on telemetry for several days, longer than you would want, because you're trying to decide, 'I've got to anticoagulate him. I may have to put a pacemaker in.' So you just buy three or four days right there, and then you commit to either accept the rhythm or put in a pacemaker, and that's not assuming any pulmonary or renal problems. I would say when he goes in for that reoperation, knowing what you're going to have to do for that to get the homograft out, you would tell the patient, and if you are going to have a complication, the most likely one other than bleeding is going to be the need for a pacemaker.

He said that needing a pacemaker was more than 51% likely. The doctor continued regarding the basis for the probability being at least 51%.

Dr. Shuman: The fact that he has had scarring in the area of his prior abscess, that you're going to have to cut out the homograft to put in the new prosthetic conduit, and that that is going to be very near the conduction system, and so quite probable that a pacemaker will be needed.

He said that in his own practice, which did not include homografts, the redo valves were 2% but the redo coronaries were more common.

201

Then Dr. Shuman added his own notes about two articles he mentioned.

Dr. Shuman: It says mortality rate, 7.5. Five-year survival, 87.3. Ten-year survival, 70.8%. Reoperations in 10.8%. The mortality rate for reoperations was 28.6%. The likelihood of endocarditis in the homografts was 3.2%. The mean follow-up was 5.8 years.

He also said that surgery is required in 50% of valvular endocarditis cases. Continuing, he said that it depends on a whole host of factors including: valve normal or abnormal, organism hospital acquired or community acquired, diagnosis made quickly or delayed, how bad the organism is, the patient himself in terms of IV drug use, AIDS, and a competent immune system.

Shuman said that depending on all those things, not everyone who develops endocarditis needs surgery. He said, by and large, it's about 50% of all diagnosed cases of endocarditis that need surgery.

If it's a *Strep* endocarditis, a surgeon may not be called at all. With *Staphylococcus,* a surgeon will be called just in case.

Mr. Ryan: Do a higher percentage of patients go on to surgery when there's *Staphylococcus aureus* involved?

Dr. Shuman: Yes.

Mr. Ryan: Greater than 50%, correct?

Dr. Shuman: Again, it all depends. Again, is it hospital-acquired, is it someone who has an in-dwelling IV catheter and he gets hospital-acquired *Staphylococcus* that tends to be more resistant. If it's community-acquired, presumably this occurred, and it may have been related to that hiking that he did. He may have scratched himself. That may have been the mechanism of getting the *Staphylococcus* in the bloodstream. That and his overall clinical course in this gentleman. **If it had been picked up appropriately, he should not have required surgery.**

Mr. Ryan: *Staphylococcus aureus* is one of the most virulent organisms that cause endocarditis, correct?

Mr. Berger: Objection. Incomplete hypothetical.

Mr. Ryan: Are there more virulent organisms that cause endocarditis on a community-acquired basis than *Staphylococcus aureus*?

Mr. Berger: Same objection.

Dr. Shuman: Yes. Fungal, *Candida*. There are other gram-negative organisms that can be very lethal.

Dr. Shuman added that if the *Staphylococcus aureus* is hospital-acquired, it is usually considered quite bad. If it is community-based, he said, it might not be bad at all.

Mr. Ryan: By hospital-acquired, you're talking about MRSA?

Dr. Shuman agreed and added that some forms of community-acquired *Staphylococcus aureus* can be more aggressive than others.

Dr. Shuman: There was nothing in the records that I saw that would indicate that his valve was anything but normal. I saw nothing in the records to indicate that he had prior AI (aortic insufficiency).

Then Dr. Shuman made one telling statement.

Dr. Shuman: But remember, he is a big guy. I think he was six-four, 265 pounds. **He is going to have a heart that is larger than most (people) simply because of his size.**

Mr. Ryan asked that everything after "remember" be stricken from Dr. Shuman's answer as nonresponsive.

Nevertheless, the damage was done as far as Ray Brinkman's testimony about my enlarged heart was concerned. It was bogus as far as being long-term or chronic, according to Dr. Shuman. And the law would have allowed such testimony at trial.

Mr. Ryan brought to the attention of all that in Dr. Soltero's notes; Dr. Soltero said that my aortic insufficiency was "probably chronic."

Dr. Shuman, under questioning, said that he had no idea why Dr. Soltero would say that about my condition, based upon the evidence that Dr. Shuman had reviewed.

Dr. Shuman said that in order to have chronic aortic insufficiency, you need to measure the heart at two different times such as now and a year earlier via echocardiograms. Since that was not the case with me, how could there be chronic aortic insufficiency noted? Plus, there was no diastolic murmur. To make a diagnosis of that without the two measurements and the murmur would be below the expected standard of care.

Dr. Shuman said that a diastolic murmur might be hard to detect depending upon the degree of intensity and the degree of training or past experience of the person listening for it. He said that there are times when some medical personnel will hear that kind of murmur and others will not.

Let me add that if you have a case where a diastolic murmur may give a clue or provide further information for a diagnosis, the last thing that you want is for a medical professional with a hearing problem to listen for it. Especially for the lower range of sounds. That is where the sounds of such a murmur would fall, in the lower decibel range.

Mr. Ryan: With mild chronic aortic insufficiency, is it true that there may not be a diastolic murmur at all because the heart adapts over time to that condition?

Dr. Shuman: No. I would say there would be a murmur.

About the pathology report on my heart valve, Shuman said that it was a normal trileaflet valve with no longstanding problems that simply was infected.

Dr. Shuman said that when a medical person talks about endocarditis, acute endocarditis is from two to three weeks or less and that chronic endocarditis is longer than two to three weeks.

Dr. Shuman felt that the endocarditis of my heart was present on March 28th. He believed that my symptoms began on March 27th. He said that to clinically confirm endocarditis, you would need a fever, positive culture, an echocardiogram and the presence of a diastolic murmur — *all four*. He said that you can have a very high suspicion of endocarditis without the murmur and echocardiogram.

Mr. Ryan asked Dr. Shuman about the significance of a vegetative growth greater than one centimeter.

Dr. Shuman said that if the vegetative growth is greater than one centimeter, the incidence of strokes or pulmonary embolisms is much, much higher than growths less than one centimeter. Above a one centimeter growth, the probability of surgery is much greater. **He said with a four-plus reading for aortic regurgitation, a dilated left ventricle, three-centimeter vegetation, a previous stroke or multiple strokes, that any of those would be clear indications for surgery.**

Dr. Shuman said that the Levaquin did its job as far as getting the *Staphylococcus aureus* under control because the cultures were negative on the 15th, 16th, 17th and 20th. In other words, forty-eight to seventy-two hours after the IV Levaquin was administered, the virulent organism was toast. **He also noted that once the virulent strain of *Staphylococcus aureus* was gone, I had another bacterium on my heart valve that was also resistant to penicillin-based antibiotics.**

In essence, I had gotten the two for one deal at Bacteria Depot.

He said that with the available evidence, if I had been placed on the appropriate antibiotic on the 30th, I would not have needed valve surgery. Further, Shuman said if that had happened, the worst case is that I would have had very mild aortic insufficiency or none. He said that on the final report for the culture, it said, "**Rare Staphylococcus species**."

In this case, the "Rare Staphylococcus Species" was a strain of *Staphylococcus areus: Staphylococcus spp. agglutinin neg.*

In a 1990 article,[xv] the authors noted how rare pathogenic coagulese-negative staphylococci (CNS) are, even though some other strains of CNS are very common. They do rear their heads, metaphorically, in cases of prosthetic valve endocarditis (PVE) and in a very small percentage of cases of native valve endocarditis (NVE). Usually, the coagulese-negative staphylococci were most commonly associated with *Staphylococcus epidermidis* and not *Staphylococcus Aureus.*

Staphylococcus spp. agglutinin neg is a coagulese-negative staphylococci.

My case involved native valve endocarditis, making mine a rare case.

He said that necrosis of the heart was caused by the organism, in that it ate away part of the valve and that there was an abscess of pus, too. Dr.

Shuman said that if the abscess had traveled into the left ventricle of my heart, it could have been a horrendous problem. He said that the presence of the necrosis and the abscess were functions of the virulence of the organism, not how long it had been there. The doctor said that if my blood could not have been made sterile by the antibiotics, surgery was a necessity. He said that you would only be able to determine when the abscess began by picking it up on an echo. Robert L. Shuman did not know when the vegetation on my heart valve started and said an echo would have shown that, if one was taken day-by-day until it showed up just like the abscess.

In summary, Dr. Shuman said I did not have pre-existing valvular heart disease. If the proper antibiotic had been administered by the 30th, surgery would not have been required. He said that this was probably the case on the 6th — that if I had been admitted on that date and the correct antibiotic administered no surgery. Shuman said that the durability of the homograft was not as great as had been hoped for in this country. He said a one centimeter growth of vegetation alone was not enough to require surgery but that with confirming signs, yes. The doctor said the risk of a stroke or embolism with a vegetative growth above one centimeter was 5%.

At that point, Dr. Shuman had finished educating all those in the room about my case and about *Staphylococcus aureus* endocarditis.

*****

DEPOSITION OF PATRICK JOSEPH, MD

Patrick Joseph, MD was hired by the defense team for Dr. Andrews to be an expert in the areas of causation and damages. He was deposed by Richard T. Lobl on Friday August 5, 2005 in Los Angeles, California. Patricia Daehnke of Bonne, Bridges, Mueller, O'Keefe and Nichols was there for defendant Raymond Arthur Andrews, MD.

Dr. Joseph stated that he had been deposed seventy-five times in the course of his career with 90% of them being taken in medical negligence cases. Of those, 65% were for the defense.

Mr. Lobl: What I'd like you to do first, if you would, is to list those opinions you have formulated regarding causation in this case.

Dr. Joseph: The opinions that I have in this case are many, but I think there's only one or two that are controversial that I think I will be asked to express in trial.

And it's my understanding that as this case has evolved, the biggest question being posed to me has to do with the effect of antibiotics provided to Mr. Folck regarding avoiding surgery. And it's my opinion that if Mr. Folck had been admitted to the hospital on the morning of April 6, 2004 and started on intravenous antibiotics that were effective against the organism recovered from his bloodstream on March 28th, that he still would have required valvular surgery to replace his aortic valve and that, since he was fortunate enough to have a relatively uncomplicated course, his condition would be the same today.

Mr. Lobl: What other opinions have you formulated regarding causation?

Dr. Joseph: Implicit in that opinion would, of course, be that if he were admitted at any time after April 6th, that the course would have been the same.

The other comment I need to address is on March 30th, since it is the first time that Dr. Andrews saw this patient, and on March 30th, it is very difficult to be certain if surgery would have been necessary, if for some reason he had received aggressive therapy. But considering the way this organism has been acting, I think that it is more probable than not that surgery would still be necessary, but I can't say it with a great deal of assuredness as I can on April 6th. I think on March 30th, it's very difficult in an honest way to make a decision about the need for surgery if antibiotics had been started.

Dr. Joseph went on to say that he believed my heart valve was infected on March 28th with a growth of staphylococci that was essentially untreated for nine days. He added that the Biaxcin which Andrews prescribed would not have been correct for the condition.

He continued saying that the organism grows to about one centimeter in seven to ten days. He said that when the first echocardiogram was taken on April 13th, the growth was described as being greater than one centimeter. He believed that by April 6th, there was probably a growth of one centimeter and that the need for surgery is greater than 50% for persons with growths of that size. He also believed that the organism stopped growing on April 6th. He added that once I had been switched to Augmentin on April 6th, the vegetation stopped growing. In other words, although there was no objective information about any vegetation on my heart valve on April 6th, Dr. Joseph's hypothetical vegetation ceased to grow.

He later added that, in some cases, Augmentin might stop such an infection as I had. **This goes against the available evidence in my case**.

In Dr. Joseph's opinion, since this was a left side endocarditis, persons with a *Staphylococcus* infection on that side of the heart with vegetation have an extremely high incidence of requiring surgery for care.

*****

Folks, this is pure speculation and an example of how expert testimony can be used to confuse jurors involved in a med mal case.

What we do know is that two chest x-rays were taken of my chest on April 6, 2004 and that there was no indication on either x-ray of anything amiss on my heart. It was not until an x-ray on April 12, 2004, ordered by Christopher Kuhlman, MD, that any problem area on my heart was detected.

Now I ask you, how could Dr. Joseph keep a straight face as he postulated what he did?

I'm not a doctor but I do have common sense.

*****

DEPOSITION OF LAWRENCE ALAN MAY, MD

Dr. May gave his deposition for my side on Wednesday August 10, 2005. Richard T. Lobl was there for me, and Patricia Daehnke was there for defendant Raymond Arthur Andrews, MD.

Because this deposition was taken so late in the case, I did not read it until I was researching this book in 2007.

Ms. Daehnke was very testy in her early questioning of Dr. May as if she wanted to catch him in a lie or misstatement or omission so as to discredit him at trial. He called her on it in the first few minutes of the deposition. She tried to accomplish the goal in a playful way and then the real questioning started.

Ms. Daehnke: How do you define the standard of care?

Dr. May: I think it's a legal definition, and I don't — I don't want to provide a legal definition. The standard of care is the expectation that a patient should have in seeing a physician, expecting a certain level of knowledge and application of that knowledge.

Ms. Daehnke: But is that the standard upon which you — to which you hold Dr. Andrews in this case?

Dr. May: I don't hold — I hold him to a standard of what I think a reasonable average physician should do in the office setting seeing a patient with complaints and history that any patient has that is being reviewed.

Dr. May went on to discuss what he thought were breaches in the standard of care by Raymond Arthur Andrews in handling my case.

Dr. May: I think that, in summary, the care fell below the standard on several occasions. And without offering opinion as to causation, I think it was contributory to an adverse outcome.

The first encounter was on March 29th (he meant March 30th).

Stated simply, Dr. May felt that Dr. Andrews did not ask enough probing questions, especially since he did not ask about me seeing any other doctor recently to get a relevant history.

Ms. Daehnke: Ok.

Dr. May: On that encounter, I think there was a failure to obtain relevant history, to obtain the relevant documentation that occurred, a failure to follow up on this history that — I don't know whether it was obtained at all or just failed to follow through on, but failure to get relevant information that would have been important to the proper care of a patient.

Ms. Daehnke: What else?

Dr. May: Well, the interaction that would generally reveal; that is, that you ask the patient. When did the symptoms begin? What have you done about the symptoms? Have you seen anyone? Have you received any care? And that would ultimately reveal an event of that importance, that the day before (actually two days) he was seen in the Emergency Room.

So, I don't know for a fact that he (Andrews) was told that. I don't know for a fact that he (Andrews) knew that. I am saying that he should have.

Ms. Daehnke seemed like a dim bulb asking how Andrews should have done that.

Mr. Lobl: I thought he just testified to that.

Ms. Daehnke kept pressing and Dr. May repeated himself several times.

Ms. Daehnke: So, your assumption is that those questions weren't asked?

Dr. May: Well, I have two assumptions to make. Either they weren't asked — assuming he (Andrews) didn't know, let's say, because I know that's his (Andrews') position that he didn't know.

Ms. Daehnke: It's also the plaintiff's position, if you read his deposition and his request or his answers to discovery responses. But go on.

Mr. Lobl: That's a misstatement.

Dr. May: I didn't read his responses to discovery. I only read his deposition, and I reflected on one question which did not lead me to know whether he (Folck) said, "No, I didn't tell him." And it's very hard to prove a negative.

Ms. Daehnke: So, Dr. Andrews should have elicited information from Mr. Folck that he had been seen in the ER?

Dr. May: Correct.

Dr. May kept hammering home the theme that Dr. Andrews, in not so many words, did not do enough to get a full picture of what had transpired with me medically between the time the blood culture was drawn and my seeing him on March 30th.

Then Lobl, Ms. Daehnke and Dr. May kicked around the subject of what Dr. Friedland knew about my having had a blood culture drawn and who ordered it and who knew the results and when the results were known.

As I read it, I realized that Ms. Daehnke was trying to direct the spotlight off her client and on to anyone remotely close to the case, specifically Dr. May and Dr. Friedland.

Dr. May offered that he believed Dr. Friedland had me go to the ER for a knee tap and that Morton ordered the blood culture on his own.

How this was relevant to Dr. Andrews' standard of care escapes me.

Dr. May once again said he felt that it was Dr. Andrews' responsibility as my primary care physician to have elicited responses from me that would have lead him to obtain all records of my ER visit on March 28th.

Ms. Daehnke: And do you have an opinion as to whether — why don't you tell me your opinion about April 6th as to whether or not Dr. Andrews met or breached the standard of care on April 6th in his care and treatment of Mr. Folck.

Dr. May: On April 6th, there are several issues that one would consider breached the standard of care. One is the relatively short shrift of a patient who's now been sick for a week with persistent fever, with no response to the Biaxcin and apparently getting sicker and is febrile in his office during the day.

The second is that after having seen him, then the patient went to the Emergency Room again. And the Emergency Room on this occasion did contact Dr. Andrews.

Dr. May basically said that Andrews took everyone else's word for what was going on with me. May offered up that Andrews never ordered any of my records from the ER visit of the 6th (by his own admission under deposition), that he relied on the opinions of others as to whether or not I needed to be hospitalized, that he did not ask me to take another blood culture when he thought the original blood culture finding might be the result of a contaminant, that, medically speaking, *Staphylococcus aureus* has a very, very low probability of being a contaminant, that my white blood count was very high with a preponderance of bands (**meaning I had a significant infection and not routine bronchitis**), disregarding the sensitivity of the blood culture and the resistance to Augmentin when that information was available, and that I should have been admitted for IV therapy with a drug like IV Levaquin.

As Dr. May put it, "He (Andrews) failed to get the actual information and failed to respond to the information available" to my detriment.

Dr. May had one last thing to say about the contaminant.

Dr. May: And I don't believe Dr. Fujita's deposition suggests that he told Dr. Andrews there was a contaminant!

*****

Other experts gave depositions, and I thank them for their input, but I only chose four medical experts to illustrate how different, in many ways, competing opinions of medical experts can be. It is not my intent to hide any deposed testimony, or to slant the case but to give you a feeling for what a jury might have to contend with. Also, space limitations do not permit summaries from every expert.

I ask you this question: *Given what you have read, how would you find in a case like mine if you were a juror knowing what you know at this point?*

Chapter 14—A Sleight of Hand

Backtracking in time just a bit, as the month of July 2005 began, Lobl and I continued to be disenchanted with one another. Every time I saw or spoke to him, he indicated how difficult a trial would be. And I kept saying that I wanted everything to come out in open court.

I also said that if the defendants were smart, they wouldn't go to trial. Lobl said that if they did settle out of court, they would expect a discount from what a jury might offer.

I looked up each and every item that Dr. Shuman said I would need as far as the future surgery and future care and after several days I arrived at a figure of $550,000. This was based on deposed testimony and the bills I had pertaining to my surgery. My estimate included one future heart valve surgery and replacement of the aortic root.

I told the amount to Rick Lobl and he said, "That would be a best case scenario."

I said, "It might be higher. I could possibly need two future heart valve surgeries."

He said, **"The insurance companies will pay for one. They won't pay for one for you when you're in your seventies!"** He spoke those words as if they were the gospel truth.

His reasons were always the same for not wanting to go to trial: the case was too difficult for a jury; I had not been fully compliant; the exact date when I could have avoided surgery was not a slam dunk; their expert witnesses would confuse the jury; etc.

You've seen the evidence. Would you agree with that assessment?

A couple times when I was in Lobl's office, we engaged in a mock question and answer about how the symptoms of the infection changed over time. I remember answering his hypothetical question about how I felt between March 28th and April 12th saying that I felt worse as time went on and then he jumped down my throat saying, "You can't say that! The defense will use that against us! They'll say you had a pre-existing condition!"

213

His comment left me very confused because what I told Lobl was true. Every time I brought something up, he took the opposite side and blew it up in my face. His favorite saying was "They're going to bring up a lot of crap."

This was the same attorney who, after going over some of my records with me *before* taking my case, said that, by the evidence in the records, he could prove negligence medical malpractice. It was disconcerting.

*****

Lobl and I got into a strictly by mail correspondence. I made sure to get everything Lobl was saying to me in writing.

In his July 5, 2005 letter to me, Rick Lobl wanted to name Dr. Friedland in the lawsuit. His reasoning was that Friedland testified in his deposition that he could not recall any interaction with Dr. Morton or anyone else at VHMC when he was informed by Morton of the positive blood culture results by Morton. This was what Dr. Morton said happened and, as such, Lobl put more credence on Morton's version of the incident.

Am I the only one who found that posturing odd?

Lobl said that the other defendants expected Friedland to be named. Rick also said that Dr. Friedland did not recall requesting me to go have my knee tapped and drained at the ER. He went on to say that if Friedland was not named as a defendant in the suit that the potential existed for the jury to find Dr. Friedland responsible, either partly or in full for my subsequent injuries. Lobl added that the risks of not naming Dr. Friedland were small, but they did exist.

I said "no" about naming Dr. Friedland.

According to Lobl, Friedland's attorney did say that Friedland would agree to a $30,000 payment but no more. I nixed it as I explained that I had had a long and beneficial relationship with Dr. Friedland and I wanted to continue that.

In a second letter dated July 5, 2005, Lobl wrote that he was disappointed that I had not given him permission to settle my case out-of-court for $400,000. He said that what I expected was too high.

Folks, Lobl had no such settlement deal with the defendants. With my approval at that figure, he would have searched for one.

He pointed out that during mediation the defendants had said that they regarded the jury verdict potential to be $450,000.

That was the first I had ever read what the defendants thought about the value of my case. At the time I read it, I felt that Lobl was lying. He wrote that with a $400,000 settlement, I would receive about $280,000.

He went on to write that things would get more expensive from then on and that I would have to foot some of the costs of the discovery and the trial.

He asked me to deposit $25,000 into a trust account for future trial expenses no later than July 22, 2005.

He also wrote that I had the right to seek new counsel if I chose to do so.

*****

I wrote back to Lobl on July 6, 2005. I asked him if my case was all smoke and mirrors, as I tried to pin him down in my letter for the date that it was a certainty that I would need an aortic valve replacement. I asked him if it was before March 28th or was it March 30th or was it some other date.

I was **explicit in my demand**, telling him that I wanted the testimony of an expert physician for our side as to what that date was. Not a best guess from the evidence on his part, but a date that could be substantiated by the available evidence.

I said, "Before I make any more decisions, I need that answer or I need to know the reason that it cannot be determined."

I told him in the letter, in not so many words, that I wasn't buying the number the defense put up since they did not say how they arrived at that number.

Lastly I wrote, **"Please let me know if you have any personal/professional conflicts that are going to interfere with my case."**

*****

Lobl wrote back on July 7, 2005 with his version of how the case would come down. It was his opinion only. He said that we were now entering the phase of expert discovery and that we would have an opinion soon.

Knowing that Mr. Lobl did not have a crystal ball, I did not put much credence in what he thought. I wanted some meat to bite into.

He said that he had retained an economist who stated that economic damages amounted to a present value of $200,000, with non-economic damages of $250,000. Lobl also wrote that the defense was seeking my psychiatric records from the V.A. in order to determine if my PTSD had been exacerbated as much as I was claiming.

I never saw the information from Lobl's economist.

I later threw in the towel on trying to recover any damages for exacerbation of my PTSD, even though I knew that it had happened. But it would have been difficult to go through at trial. So I cut it loose.

Lobl further wrote that a plaintiff's verdict was 75% likely in my case although, statistically, juries found in favor of a physician about 80% of the time.

*****

In my response letter, I got down and dirty about settling for $400,000. I wrote back on July 10, 2005 asking him, **"Is your firm in financial difficulty? Are you protecting any of the defendants from a large potential verdict? Would a large verdict make it difficult to work with these defendants in the future? Does your firm not have the finances to carry this case through trial? What are you not telling me that might make me want to consider a minor settlement? Why am I supposed to suffer a future hardship to appease the defense?"**

I continued on with "If you answer 'yes' to any of the questions above or you are unwilling to give me a straight answer, you need to consider excusing yourself as counsel."

I continued with **"I see a huge conflict between you and your past association with Harold Morton in this case."**

He responded that, basically, everything was fine, that there was no conflict, that things were moving forward and that he was not protecting anyone.

Thinking about it now, it's possible that Lobl did this sort of thing frequently; that is, bandy about numbers during the course of a case. In his world, you started somewhere, you ended up somewhere else. He knew it wasn't gospel when he started but I didn't. It was like dickering with a car salesman in the old days. And it drove me crazy.

In my world, when you are talking about serious financial stuff and the numbers keep changing, it's like **"The Big Lie."** It meant that someone was lying to me and I got turned off by it very quickly.

In my mind, my medical case value was not like the price of a car that changed during negotiations, but that is how it felt. One time I got one number, another time another number.

Around this time in my case, I was wearing down emotionally, and it didn't help that I was not feeling like I was getting straight answers from Lobl. Also, I was very concerned about money and my future since, technically, I no longer had a job with Farmers Insurance. That thought was beating on me. What the hell was I going to do about that?

217

I wondered if I might be getting set up by my own attorney because of some things he had told me in his office prior to taking my case. But was that really the case?

I was so concerned that I wrote to Judge John Farrell, the presiding judge in the case, but the letters I sent to him were returned. Apparently, I could not contact the Judge by letter.

I was anxious, depressed, and uncertain and I was a mess emotionally as time went on. That was nothing new for me. It was just getting higher and deeper.

*****

As part of the pre-trial process, a mandatory out-of-court settlement conference in the Judge's chambers is required. The Judge assigned to the case tries to wield his considerable influence to get a settlement.

On Monday August 1, 2005 at about 9:45 am, I sat on a bench in the area outside Department F49 at the Superior Court for the County of Los Angeles in Chatsworth, California. My turn before the Judge was close at hand.

Michael Berger was there. Rick Lobl was in Colorado chasing down a potential case that turned out later to be bogus. I wish that I had picked up the clue that money might be a problem in Lobl's office, since he spent money chasing a bogus case. At least, that is what I thought years later.

Dr. Andrews was waiting there outside the Superior Court with his attorney. Harold Morton did not show up there, but a lawyer for him did. Also in the area was a lawyer from VHMC and a person high up in the hospital administration.

Dr. Andrews' female attorney, Patricia Daehnke, walked up to me. She introduced herself. We shook hands and exchanged small talk. Then she said, "Well, it was very nice meeting you," and then she walked away.

*****

At 10:00 am, everyone was called into the courtroom. Judge John Farrell was presiding. Everyone was called to order. The Judge spoke for a couple of minutes and then called the attorneys into his chambers.

I sat in the courtroom. Dr. Andrews was also there. He had his eyes tightly closed and he looked like he was praying. His head was tilted down and his hands were clasped together.

*****

More than 90 minutes later, everyone came out of the Judge's chambers and back into the courtroom.

Dr. Andrews and his attorney scurried out of the courtroom. On their way out, Dr. Andrews said to his attorney, "I didn't do anything!"

I thought, "That's for damn sure!"

Michael Berger sat next to me and said, "The Judge asked but did not order all parties to return to this courtroom at 1:30 pm today. There was a lot of finger-pointing in the Judge's chambers as to who was guilty and who didn't do what. They really went after each other. You wouldn't believe what they said to each other!"

I drove home and had lunch while I contemplated my next move.

*****

At 1:30 pm, Judge William Farrell, Judge John Farrell's older brother, appeared on the bench. Raymond Andrews and his attorney were not present. They never returned to court that day.

219

Judge Farrell was irritated that they were not in the courtroom. He waited about ten minutes before speaking.

He said, "My brother, the other Judge Farrell, is trying to settle another civil matter and it is at a very sensitive stage. So he asked me to appear. Since I had nothing on the docket for this afternoon, I agreed to be here."

He made a couple of remarks and said, "From what I know about this case, Dr. Andrews has some serious issues to get resolved in the care and treatment of the defendant. He should be here with counsel."

I asked if I could say something. The Judge said that it was fine for me to speak.

I reminded the Judge that I had been a juror in the Superior Court in Van Nuys in a trial he had presided over. I reminded him of the case.

Judge William Farrell said that he remembered the case, and we had a short and pleasant conversation on the record. I got the feeling that by bonding with the Judge over that past case, there was a good chance that he would make sure there was no underhandedness regarding this possible settlement.

Deciding to wait no longer for Andrews and his attorney, Judge John Farrell summoned all parties to his chambers to resume settlement negotiations.

I later learned that during the lunch recess, Lobl had spoken with Michael Berger via telephone from Colorado. Lobl told Berger that he felt I should settle with the hospital and Dr. Morton, and that we should go to trial against Dr. Andrews. Lobl bandied about a figure of $250,000 to Berger.

Lobl said the trial would be for "cause." This meant, under the law, that even if Dr. Andrews was only found to be 1% liable for his negligence, he would be on the hook for the entire difference between the jury verdict and what was paid out-of-court from the hospital and Dr. Morton.

Hypothetically, let's say a $550,000 jury verdict was rendered, and an out-of-court settlement for $300,000 was reached with all the other defendants. Andrews would then owe $250,000. So, by putting his side in a situation where a finding of "cause" was possible because Andrews and his attorney did not return for the afternoon session, the non-settling defendant could cause the amount his carrier might have to shell out to be more than what they anticipated.

*****

About twenty minutes later, Michael Berger came out of the Judge's chambers, and he told me what Rick Lobl had told him. I let it sink in. I gave it a few moments to swirl around in my head.

After a brief pause, Michael Berger added, ***"Rick says that a trial will cost $20,000."***

I asked, "Is he sure about that?"

Berger said, **"Yes, he used that figure several times."**

I thought some more.

Berger said, "You have a very good case for 'cause' against Dr. Andrews. If you settle with Dr. Morton, Dr. Fujita will testify against Dr. Andrews."

My deliberations in this matter took about ten minutes in total.

I said, "Ok, let's go for it. But $250,000 for the two of them is too low. And as long as the trial costs $20,000."

Michael Berger said, "You're right. I'll get more. **And the trial will cost $20,000.**" With that, he went back into the Judge's chambers.

Then the lawyers negotiated however lawyers negotiate. I waited while they did their lawyering.

*****

At 4:00 pm that day, two out-of-court settlements were reached in the case — one with VHMC and one with Harold Morton, MD. The Judge called the court to order and asked me a requisite list of questions to determine if I knew what the settlement amount was, what I was agreeing to, was I of sound mind at this time, etc. Judge Farrell said that I had a strong case against Dr. Andrews. He also said that I had been ably represented by Mr. Berger. The Judge referred to him as a very good attorney.

According to the settlement agreement, I could not disclose the amount.

Judge William Farrell said, "All parties must return to the courtroom two weeks from today."

*****

Two weeks after agreeing to a partial out-of-court settlement, all the necessary parties reconvened before Judge John Farrell.

Rick Lobl sat next to me in Department F49. Lobl casually asked me if I indeed wanted a partial out-of-court settlement. I said that I did.

In his hand, Lobl had a response to a 998 demand letter sent to Dr. Andrews' attorney asking for an out-of-court settlement from Dr. Andrews through his insurance carrier. Lobl handed me the letter and said, "Maybe you will see something before trial."

The gist of their response to the "998 letter" was that they might consider settling if the amount was below the lower amount the two settling defendants agreed to settle for. One paid more, one paid less than the other.

Judge John Farrell, the first Judge Farrell, asked me the requisite questions once again. Satisfied with my answers, he ordered the settlement with VHMC and Dr. Morton finalized and the legally agreed amounts to be paid to Mr. Lobl who would make my disbursement.

The people representing the hospital apologized to me for what had happened. So did Dr. Morton's attorney. I said that I had been pushed into a corner about this and, because that was the case, I saw no other avenue than to file suit.

With that, I left the courthouse.

*****

Three days later, I got a call from Rick Lobl's office. The person speaking to me said that I could pick up my check and that Rick wanted to speak to me about the trial costs against Dr. Andrews.

When I got to Lobl's office, everything was in order, I understood the breakdown of costs that had to be paid to Lobl, **but the check was $35,000 short of what I expected**. I asked him, "What happened to the $35,000?"

He said that $35,000 was being withheld for upcoming trial expenses against Dr. Andrews. He said that, in reality, the case against Dr. Andrews would cost $35,000. He further added that the case against Dr. Andrews was not that good and that he needed the extra money in reserve in case he had some additional expenses to prove the case. I let it all sink in.

I looked at my check less the $35,000 and said that by accepting the money, I had given up my rights at trial for "cause" verdicts against the hospital and/or Dr. Morton. And that they were clearly more liable than Andrews.

Without missing a beat, Lobl said, **"Your case was not that good to begin with!** You're fortunate to be getting any money at all, especially since Harold Morton ordered the blood culture that disclosed the *staphylococcus* infection."

Can you believe that?! I felt dumbfounded and I was reeling. It took balls to say that.

The reality was that Morton failed miserably!

Lobl said, "I can get you $30,000 right now to settle out-of-court against Andrews. I am good friends with the Vice-President of his malpractice insurance company who has the purse strings for his case. Just say the word and I'll make a call."

He added that the friendship he had with the insurance carrier executive was purely social. He said that he and his wife had enjoyed the company of the executive and her husband on a number of occasions.

I had asked him in a letter if he had any personal or professional relationships that would interfere with him representing me.

I had written the letter because some things about the progression of the case were not adding up in my mind. He had replied, in writing, that he did not have any conflicting relationships. These letters were exchanged before any settlement before the Judge was even offered. Had he said "yes," I would have dropped him *on the spot*.

What he said didn't hit me until I got home.

Do any of you think that Lobl was playing **God**?

Only a couple weeks earlier, Lobl had told Michael Berger to tell me that the cost of a trial against Dr. Andrews was $20,000 (at the time when we were negotiating for an out-of-court settlement).

Folks, we got into a major beef over this, let me tell you.

*****

I called Lobl's office from home the next day and said that I wanted the $35,000. I told his office person to tell him that I did not authorize him to keep that money.

I heard part of a muffled conversation in the background and then heard Rick Lobl shout, at the top of his voice, "If you keep that money, you can get yourself another attorney!"

Was Lobl revealing his desperation for money to keep his practice going?

I recalled that when I was discussing the case with Rick Lobl, he told me that the case in which Dr. Morton had testified on behalf of Rick's client was a case where Dr. Morton testified as an expert witness on infectious diseases of the bloodstream! That's right, **Harold Morton knew MRSA and sensitivities to antibiotics like he knew the back of his own hand but he had played that down in my case**.

I said to the person from Lobl's office, "Get my check ready, I'm on my way over." With that, I hung up.

Had I been played by Rick Lobl?

I was so upset as to not utter a word. At a time when a celebration should have been in the offing, his maneuvering was a major downer.

Had the out of court settlement been a sham to protect Morton more than to help me?

Was Lobl willing to sell me out to Andrews' carrier where he had a social friend who was an executive?

I thought of two words: "Closed club."

I was irate.

Like a combat soldier facing great bodily harm or death, I was in a mode to "take as many of them down with me" as I could if I was going down.

This was war!

*****

I went to Lobl's office to pick up the check for $35,000. Michael Berger showed me some papers that Rick wanted me to sign releasing Rick as my attorney. I refused to sign them. I got my check and left.

A couple of days later, I got papers in the mail from Rick's office to sign to drop him as my attorney. I didn't sign them.

Then Lobl filed a NOTICE OF MOTION AND MOTION TO BE RELIEVED AS COUNSEL (in late August 2005) with the court requesting that he be allowed to drop me as a client. He stated that the relationship between us was irrevocably broken beyond repair (or words to that effect) and that I had not followed the retainer agreement (which was true) by not advancing money to Lobl when he requested it. I was not going to shell out any more money to Lobl.

I responded to Mr. Lobl's motion and filed my own motion with the court acting as my own attorney. In not so many words, I told the court that even though I probably needed an attorney to help settle the remainder of the case, I could no longer trust Richard T. Lobl because he had misled me as to how much a trial against Dr. Andrews would cost ($35,000 instead of $20,000) and that he had changed his story as to what kind of a case I had against Dr. Andrews. Because I was misled, I had settled out-of-court against the two other defendants in the case.

At the end of my declaration, I said, "After detailing some of the problems I have had with Mr. Lobl's representation in this case so far, I do not oppose his withdrawal as my counsel. I cannot have an attorney represent me whom I do not trust in such a serious matter."

Lobl responded in court documents that the actual trial cost would be closer to $20,000. I guess he felt he had to get that on the record for whatever reason. Maybe it was a last ditch effort to save his reputation. If word of this got out, his word would be worthless. He later denied this to The State Bar of California.

To me, **I thought nothing could be better than to make public how he tried to up the trial cost on me and jack me around.**

I did not show up for the hearing and Lobl was relieved as my counsel by order of the court.

*****

According to *U.S. News—Best Lawyers®*, Richard T. Lobl is ranked as a Tier 1 attorney (with 1 being best) both in Los Angeles and Nationally.

I couldn't agree less with those rankings.

At that moment the idea that maybe a Ouija board had been used to evaluate Lobl came to mind.

*****

Emotionally, I was toast. I was crackers. All the stress, the disappointment, the betrayal, the deceit!

I searched for about a week for another attorney to represent me. I remember one medical malpractice attorney in Van Nuys in particular who reviewed my case. His name was Nick Kazandjieff. I thought Nick was very competent and a straight shooter.

Nick and the other med mal attorneys mostly said the same thing: The case had been gutted, and there was not enough money left in it to warrant them preparing for a trial. Others said that they couldn't understand why I even sued in the first place. One asked me, "What does a blood *Staphylococcus* infection have to due with an aortic valve replacment?"

Nick said that the evidence against Dr. Andrews, especially from my expert witness, Dr. Lawrence Alan May, was weak. He, like the other attorneys I contacted, was not interested in representing me and felt that I could not find one who would just conduct a deposition since so much preparation was involved.

*****

Please take note. Have all of your ducks lined up against all defendants before you head into a trial. Be clear what each expert will testify to under oath before your side designates that person as an expert or you might get sandbagged. In other words, pay a few thousand for a preliminary opinion, rather than waiting to hear what your expert will say in a deposition during the deposition — as was the case with Dr. May.

*****

With the filing of the court documents, Andrews' attorney Patricia Daehnke got wind of it. She called me. I asked Daehnke if there was any possibility of an out-of-court settlement with her client. Daehnke said that she would consider it if she could depose one of the experts on my list. In other words, she wanted to find out what she would be up against in court.

I thought about it for a couple days. I felt that I couldn't find anyone who would represent me for that.

I was up against the wall, so I signed the papers releasing Dr. Andrews as a defendant.

*****

My mouth had a caustic taste in it from the legal crap. I was major league depressed. It lasted for about four or five months. I gutted it out with every ounce of energy I could summon up. It never got to the point of suicidal ideation. Fortunately, I never tried to harm myself.

I had several walk-in visits at Building 10 on the Sepulveda V.A. Medical Center campus in North Hills, California for psychiatric consults, along with my regular visits to a psychiatric resident during those very "black" months. I went up to a clinical dosage on my main antidepressant, Effexor, of 450 mg per day to get through the really tough days.

228

I wanted to kill Lobl and Morton, metaphorically. At least I gave serious thought to harming both of them. My thought was that I was going to use a large baseball bat on both of them. It never came to fruition. I let the ugly thoughts die. A couple of times, I wanted to get an axe and chop down Lobl's office door. That way, there would be no more secrets to hide in that place!

Finally, the storm passed. I had been out of control about the whole incident for way too long. It was time to move forward.

It was time for me to blow the whistle on those who I felt were guilty of medical malpractice to the Medical Board of California.

Under California law, if a physician is involved in the settlement of a medical malpractice case, that person must be named on a report to the Medical Board of California. It is not considered a complaint. Complaints are handled differently by special investigators working for The Medical Board.

If a non-physician healthcare provider is involved in the claim or action, a report need not be filed with the Medical Board of California. However, there may be reporting requirements to other professional licensing boards or bureaus in the state.

If any of the defendants in the case was unlicensed at the time of the injury, no report needs to be made to the Medical Board of California. **Residents, interns, and medical students have not demonstrated that they have minimum entry level competence as physicians. So you cannot, under the law, sue them for medical malpractice. That is why Dr. Fujita was never sued.**

As far as the amount of the settlement is concerned, if it exceeds $30,000 a report must be made to the Medical Board of California. This encourages smaller settlements so that the guilty party avoids any punishment or license probation or suspension. All defendant physicians must be named. If no apportionment is made (regarding the award) toward a specific defendant, each and every licensed physician named as a defendant will have the entire amount reported to the Medical Board of California.

When a complaint is filed with the Medical Board of California, staff members in the Central Complaint Unit review all information to determine if a violation of the Medical Practice Act occurred. Each named physician is given an opportunity to respond. And using an attorney to respond is permissible. If a physician disagrees with the report, he is allowed to contact the person or entity who made the report to discuss it with them.

Any judgments or arbitration awards are posted upon receipt of settlement monies. Settlements resolved after 1-1-03 are disclosed by the

Medical Board of California after a physician has accumulated three or four settlements within a ten year period (depending upon the specialty of a physician).

Under "Quality of Medical Care Complaints," if the Board determines that the licensee's actions were not below the standards of acceptable care, the Board will close the complaint and do nothing. If the Board finds that the standard of care was below acceptable standards, but that it did not constitute "Gross Negligence Medical Malpractice," the complaint will be closed with no actions taken and will be kept on file. If a complaint is found to meet the standards of "Gross Negligence Medical Malpractice," the case may be submitted to the Office of the Attorney General.

What are the potential punishments or sanctions that the Medical Board of California can administer based upon the evidence in a particular case?

Among the remedies are: (1) public censure, (2) probation for a licensed medical care provider, (3) suspension of the medical care provider's license for a certain period of time, (4) revocation of a medical care provider's license, and (5) criminal prosecution.

*****

I filed two complaints with the Medical Board of California regarding my case. One was against Raymond Arthur Andrews, MD. The other was against Edward Nathan Morton, MD. Both alleged gross negligence medical malpractice on their parts in the *handling* of my *Staphylococcus aureus* infection. Actually, *mishandling* is the proper descriptive word.

A few weeks after filing against each of them, I was contacted by a female investigator from the Medical Board. I believe that she was a Senior Investigator. I remember that she was not a rookie.

The woman came to my house, and I spent two hours with her going over what had happened. She took copious notes. I showed her some of the records I had obtained and so forth. Since I had all the depositions and filings on the legal side of things, I showed those to her. She said that this was the worst case of a botched *Staphylococcus aureus* infection that she had ever investigated.

As we finished up, she asked me what I wanted to see happen to Dr. Andrews and Dr. Morton. I said, "They both need to go away from practicing medicine for a while over this."

She said that it was clear in her mind that malpractice had occurred with Dr. Morton the moment he sent me out into the night while taking Augmentin, which was a penicillin-based drug (treating a penicillin-resistant bacteria). She said that it appeared that Dr. Andrews was negligent as well. She added that she would have to review everything before making a final determination about him.

I said that I understood. I told her that I felt I needed to report these incidents so the two of them would not make the same mistakes again.

She thanked me and then left.

A couple days later, a copying service picked up all the medical files pertaining to my case. They copied them and returned the files about three days later.

*****

I'm sure that Morton and Andrews were doing hand springs while the Medical Board of California investigated my complaints against them. I was most interested to know what the State was going to do about them. I reveled in the idea that the heat was on them.

Dr. Andrews was investigated. Since he had not agreed to any settlement out-of-court, he was not punished in any way. Without that capitulation on his part, nothing happened to him. Had there been a trial verdict against him, possibly disciplinary action would have been taken.

As for Dr. Morton, that was a different story.

On November 22, 2006, a COMPLAINT was filed against Dr. Morton by THE DIVISION OF MEDICAL QUALITY, MEDICAL BOARD OF CALIFRONIA, and the STATE OF CALIFORNIA with the California Attorney General's Office. In the **FIRST CAUSE FOR DISCIPLINE** (gross negligence), it said that Dr. Morton was subject to disciplinary action under Section 2234, Subsection (b), of the Code in that he failed to diagnose and treat my blood *staphylococcus* (*staph.*) infection.

In short, it said that from all information available on April 6, 2004, I should have been hospitalized and treated with the proper antibiotic that was not penicillin-based since I had an infection involving penicillin-resistant bacteria. The failure to do that in a timely manner constituted an extreme departure from the standard of care.

In the **SECOND CAUSE FOR DISCIPLINE** (failure to maintain adequate and accurate records), Dr. Morton was subject to disciplinary action under Section 2266 of the Code in that he failed to maintain adequate and accurate records in the care and treatment of me. It went on to say that despite having access to the positive lab results in my records, there was nothing in Dr. Morton's notes or "summary" referencing that I had a positive blood culture, although it would be custom and practice for a reasonable doctor to write down this type of information.

In short, by not doing that, he violated a standard of care.

Under **PRAYER**, it said that a hearing should be held on the alleged matters, and that following the hearing, the Division of Medical Quality would issue a decision (from one of the following):

1. Revoking or suspending Physician's and Surgeon's Certificate issued to Harold E. Morton;
2. Revoking, suspending or denying approval of Harold E. Morton, MD's authority to supervise physician's assistants, pursuant to Section 3527 of the Code;
3. Ordering Harold E. Morton, MD to pay the Division of Medical Quality the costs of probation monitoring if he is placed on probation;
4. Taking such other and further action as deemed necessary and proper.

It was signed by David T. Thornton, Executive Director of the Medical Board of California.

*****

About six months later, a hearing was set in downtown Los Angeles at the State Attorney General's office to pass legal judgment on Edward Nathan Morton. I was notified and ready to testify, under oath, against Dr. Morton. At the last minute, I received a letter from the A.G.'s office which said that due to budget constraints, an out-of-court arrangement was made where Dr. Morton would keep his license but would be placed on probation.

So, some "doctor" could FUBAR your clinical diagnosis and mistreat you, medically, cause you to have your chest cut open so you could endure the most invasive, painful medical procedure, require you to have ongoing medical care for the rest of your life, and only get probation. What a system!

I called the attorney for the A.G.'s office who was handling the matter to find out what was up. He said that, legally, since a jury had not found against Dr. Morton, and the evidence was only from an out-of-court settlement, it was not as strong as evidence presented at a trial.

Remember, Dr. Morton had told Lobl that he did not want to be named and that he would **settle out-of-court** if the evidence pointed to his liability. And Lobl had pushed me into an out-of-court settlement. If I had known that Dr. Morton might only receive probation with an out of court settlement, I would have gone to trial against him.

As I looked back on this, I felt that an experienced attorney and a doctor who had seen other doctors go through malpractice cases had to know that settling out of court reduced the probability of a suspended license. I can't prove that Morton conveyed this to Lobl and that Lobl knew what Morton really meant and would act accordingly for Morton when he said he would settle. You can judge for yourself.

234

If I had taken Dr. Morton to trial and won, I probably could have gotten his license suspended. And I had hoped for that — a judgment against him and his license suspended.

*****

After considering what I felt was unjust in my mind, I summoned up the courage to call Wendy. I caught her when she had a few moments to talk. I told her how the legal part of the case had ended. About Rick Lobl, she said, **"He f—ked you over!"**

I asked her if what had happened constituted legal malpractice.

Wendy said that, all things considered, it probably didn't. However, she felt that it was highly unethical. She said that I might be able to seek some redress with a civil case against Rick Lobl. I thanked her.

I decided to file a complaint with the State Bar of California against Rick Lobl. I'm sure he was overjoyed to have them messing around in his business investigating my complaint. The combat soldier's mentality was running rampant in my head.

I alleged a "conflict of interest" and also that Lobl lured me into a settlement by telling me when I settled with Dr. Morton and VHMC that the trial cost would be $20,000. Later on, he asked me for $35,000. I also indicated that Lobl told me I had a good case against Andrews. By settling with those parties, I gave up my rights for potentially more money.

The State Bar sent me a reply dated February 27, 2007. In it, they informed me that it was not a conflict of interest to sue a person (on behalf of a client) who had previously been an expert witness for the attorney. Nor was it a conflict of interest for Lobl to take a case where he knew an executive at one of the defendant insurance companies.

They misstated the allegation about the $20,000 becoming $35,000, saying that the figure I was given by Mr. Berger from Mr. Lobl was for legal costs to date. **That was a lie.**

They obviously did not read what I had written and took Rick's word over mine. **Someone lied through his teeth.**

In the end, they did not find any evidence that Lobl violated any statutes or codes in his representation of me. So, no punishment was doled out. The State Bar said that they did not get involved in civil matters between attorneys and clients.

I learned that when you go after an attorney through the State Bar, the burden of proof has to be "**clear and convincing evidence**" (much closer to "beyond a reasonable doubt") than a mere "preponderance" of evidence, which is the usual standard of proof in civil matters.

I did not pursue a civil case against Rick Lobl. It would have been very costly, and it would have ended up being his word against mine (except for possibly some testimony from Michael Berger) in a pissing match.

I did send a letter to Lobl telling him I wanted some of his fee back that he had received under the law for the settlement. He did not respond.

*****

I was finished with my case. Actually, I was sick and tired of it. There was nothing left to do but to get on with my life.

Part III: Medical Malpractice Laws
and Reform Ideas

So again, I ask you… **Should you have your head examined before filing a medical malpractice lawsuit? Particularly, in California? This chapter takes a look at the current related laws in the Golden State.**

*****

John D. Winer, a San Francisco attorney from the law firm of Winer and McKenna, who handles plaintiffs' medical malpractice cases, provided many of the thoughts contained in this chapter. They are used with his permission.

What follows is largely an abridged version of John Winer's guide.[xvi]

This information is provided as background only. You should consult a California med mal attorney if you have questions about this state's MICRA provisions that pertain to your particular case. Consult a med mal attorney within your state for legal advice if you live outside of California.

*****

The California Medical Injury Compensation Reform Act (MICRA) of 1975 was enacted by the California State Legislature in August 1975 and signed into law in September 1975 **to limit medical malpractice insurance premiums** for California healthcare providers.

The MICRA covers legal rules involving medical malpractice actions in California, including monetary damages. It took certain kinds of tort actions out of the general legal system and put them under the heading of medical malpractice.

*****

In the view of the California State Legislature in 1975, a "crisis" existed regarding medical malpractice insurance. The rising cost of medical malpractice insurance premiums was **supposedly** imposing serious problems for the healthcare system in California.

Legislators and others believed that the crisis threatened to reduce the availability of medical care in some parts of the State. Without intervention, they felt that a very real possibility existed that many doctors would practice without insurance thus reducing the possibility that injured patients could not collect monetary damages even if they got a court judgment in their favor.

The Legislature felt that the continuing availability of adequate medical care depended directly on the availability of adequate medical malpractice insurance coverage. In their way of thinking, lower medical malpractice insurance premiums would mean that more doctors would be available to serve Californians' medical needs. This, in turn, related to the costs associated with medical malpractice litigation.

The MICRA's aim was to decrease the awards for monetary damages for non-economic damages in an effort to keep healthcare providers, as a whole, financially solvent, thus lowering the cost of healthcare services and increasing their availability to patients.

*****

Medical malpractice lawsuits are based upon a breach of a healthcare provider's duty to the patient to perform his or her duties with the skill required of similar members of the profession.

This *"standard of care"* is the key concept of medical malpractice cases.

What constitutes medical malpractice in California?

Medical malpractice, sometimes referred to as medical negligence, occurs when a healthcare provider violates the governing **standard of care** when providing treatment to a patient, causing the patient to suffer an injury. Medical malpractice can result from an action taken by the medical practitioner, or by the failure to take a medically appropriate action. Examples of medical malpractice include:

- Misdiagnosis of or failure to diagnose a disease or medical condition
- Failure to provide treatment for a medical condition
- Unreasonable delay in treating a diagnosed medical condition

Medical malpractice can be brought by the injured patient (or guardian in the case of a minor) against any responsible healthcare provider, including doctors, counselors, psychologists and psychotherapists.

In order to pursue a medical malpractice case you must show evidence that: the standard of care was violated; that violation caused an injury; have a doctor testify under oath that the injury was due to a violation of the standard of care. You must have all three elements.

What is meant by *standard of care*?

The term *standard of care* **means healthcare professionals exercise that degree of skill, knowledge and care ordinarily possessed and exercised by other members of the profession acting under similar conditions and circumstances in a similar locality.**

A practitioner will be held to a higher standard of care if he or she has specialized training, regardless of whether or not the practitioner holds himself or herself out as a specialist. Thus, for instance, a cardiothoracic surgeon must comply with a standard of care of other cardiothoracic surgeons.

A medical professional who, in the course of his or her work, conforms to an accepted standard of care cannot be held liable under The MICRA, even though the treatment proves unsuccessful.

Without a provable standard of care violation, the plaintiff has no case. This applies even if there is an error in judgement made by a defendant.

A judge will instruct jurors in medical negligence cases that a healthcare provider is not necessarily negligent because he or she errs in judgment or because his or her efforts prove unsuccessful. There is only liability if the healthcare provider failed to use reasonable care and skill in his or her application of medical learning.

A healthcare provider is charged with the responsibility to consult a specialist or refer a patient to a specialist when he or she knows, or in the exercise of reasonable care should know, that a superior treatment might thereby be obtained.

A general practitioner who does not seek or recommended a specialist's advice, when a reasonably prudent practitioner would do so and a specialist is available, will be held to the standard of care applicable to specialists in the particular area of medicine.

Who sets these standards?

The **Medical Board of California** sets the standards for acceptable medical care in the State. The standards are well-known to licensed healthcare professionals in California.

Is there a statute of limitation in medical malpractice cases?

Medical malpractice cases have their own special time limitations. The rules that establish the statute of limitations in medical malpractice cases are extremely complex and confusing.

Medical malpractice cases must be brought within *three years* after the date of the injury or *one year* after the plaintiff discovers, or through the use of reasonable diligence should have discovered, the injury, whichever occurs first.

Injury has been defined as "the damaging effect of the alleged wrongful act, rather than the wrongful act itself." This means that in some cases a plaintiff can bring a medical malpractice action long after the supposed three-year "outside" time period.

There are many cases in which an injury does not manifest itself within three years of the malpractice. For instance, the three-year statute of limitations will not bar a case in which a physician ordered a chest x-ray but failed to read the results which would have revealed a cancerous tumor and the patient did not develop any noticeable symptoms in her chest for five years. Should the plaintiff, for no apparent reason, develop chest or lung symptoms, they have a duty to do due diligence under the law to investigate to see if malpractice was the cause of these symptoms.

There are exceptions to these rules but time and space do not allow an extended discussion. Winer's guide does.

What are *"caps"* and how do they work under The MICRA?

Caps under The MICRA set a ceiling or upper limit on the amount of monetary compensation that can be paid out by law.

The MICRA caps monetary awards in medical malpractice cases at $250,000 for pain and suffering (non-economic damages). This includes past and future pain and suffering, disfigurement, and physical impairment.

Even if malpractice causes death, the plaintiff(s) can only collect $250,000. By comparison, wrongful death suits can bring millions in civil court awards.

How does California compare to other states on caps for non-economic damages?

The following chart shows the cap level for non-economic damages for every state. The date of the information used in the chart is May 15, 2013.

STATE BY STATE MEDICAL MALPRACTICE

NON-ECONOMIC DAMAGE LIMITS (CAPS)

Alabama	No limit
Alaska	$400,000
Arizona	No limit
Arkansas	No limit $250,000 for punitive damages or 3 times economic damages up to $1 million
California	$250,000
Colorado	$300,000
Connecticut	No limit
Delaware	No limit
Florida	$500,000 It is applied per claimant against practitioners and $750,000 against non-practitioners. Limits are increased to $1,000,000 and $1.5 million respectively in death cases or where patient is in a vegetative state. $150,000 limit per claimant or $300,000 for all claimants when injury occurred during emergency services
Georgia	No limit
Hawaii	$375,000
Idaho	$250,000 adjusted annually
Illinois	No limit

Indiana	$250,000 liability limit per provider and excess up to $1,000,000 funded by Patient Compensation Fund
Iowa	No limit
Kansas	$250,000 limit from all defendants by each party who sues
Kentucky	No limit
Louisiana	$500,000 total recovery limit with healthcare provider limited to $100,000. Excess award paid from Patient Compensation Fund.
Maine	No limit but wrongful death cases non-economic damages are limited to $150,000
Maryland	$650,000 from 2005-2008 and increased by $15,000 per year each year after 2008
	In 2012, the limit was $710,000 and in wrongful death cases with two or more beneficiaries, the limit was $887,500.
Massachusetts	$500,000 It is adjusted annually by state treasurer according to consumer price index change. It can be higher if certain conditions are met.
Michigan	$280,000 It can go as high as $500,000 in some cases. It is adjusted by the State Treasurer every year.
Minnesota	No limit
Mississippi	$500,000
Missouri	No limit
Montana	$250,000
Nebraska	$1,750,000 total limit on all damages and each health care provider limited to $500,000 liability with excess paid by Excess Liability Fund

Nevada	$350,000
New Hampshire	No limit
New Jersey	No limit
New Mexico	$600,000 It is a total limit with additional awards for medical expenses and punitive damages.
New York	No limit
North Carolina	$500,000 It is subject to increase every third year beginning in 2014 according to Consumer Price Index.
North Dakota	$500,000
Ohio	$250,000 up to $350,000 per plaintiff or $500,000 per occurrence but does not apply to wrongful death. For estates, pain and suffering is limited to what amount of pains and suffering patient experienced prior to death.
Oklahoma	$300,000 but no limits on negligence or wrongful death
Oregon	No limit (under most circumstances)
Pennsylvania	No limit
Rhode Island	No limit with minimum of $100,000 in wrongful death cases.
South Carolina	No limit
South Dakota	$500,000
Tennessee	No limit
Texas	$250,000 per claimant with a $500,000 limit against all healthcare institutions
Utah	$450,000 Exceptions apply pertaining to when the injury occurred.

Vermont	No limit
Virginia	$2,000,000 on acts or omissions after 7/1/2008
Washington	No limit but cannot exceed formulation of average annual wage and life expectancy of injured.
West Virginia	$250,000 and up to $500,000 in more serious cases
Wisconsin	$350,000 after May 25, 1995 adjusted annually for inflation
Wyoming	No limits

As you can see, California has the lowest caps for non-economic damages in the nation along with Montana. Other states allow for higher caps and adjustments for inflation via annual changes in the Consumer Price Index. Some states set caps for non-economic damages but have excess liability funds or patient compensation funds which will pay beyond the cap limits sometimes up to a preset limit. In some states, there are no limits either because there is no statute or because of a state Supreme Court decision in a particular state to throw out cap limits for non-economic damages.

In short, California is way behind the times and is not at all progressive in changing cap limits. The present cap limit is the biggest bone of contention about The MICRA on both sides.

The MICRA takes away the right to sue for uncapped monetary damages in an amount that is commensurate in comparable civil cases.

Plaintiffs can seek **recovery of incurred and future medical expenses** as a result of the defendant's negligence.

However, **you can't get punitive damages under The MICRA —no matter how egregious the malpractice is regarding medical treatment.** The sued medical professional and/or entity and the responsible carrier get a free pass on that. Punitive damages are possible (for intentional acts, sexual abuse, and elder abuse that occurred while patients were cared for) but not for healthcare reasons.

The **MICRA reduces the consequences of bad medical care by reducing monetary damages against guilty defendants.** The defendants don't pay but their insurers do. So, it never hits them directly in their wallets. It leaves the victims of such bad medical care wanting. It also provides no incentive for medical care providers to individually or collectively weed out dangerous medical care providers. It is strictly a reactionary system, not a preventative system for future malpractice errors.

How are plaintiffs' attorneys fees calculated?

Attorneys' contingency fees in medical malpractice cases are limited under the Business and Professions Code Section 6146. In all other types of injury suits (except where the plaintiff is a minor), the parties are free to negotiate a contingency fee agreeable to all. In general, these fees are 33 1/3% of any settlement before any suit is filed and 40% after the suit has been filed.

The MICRA caps attorney fees as follows:

- 40% of the first $50,000
- 33.3% of the next $50,000
- 25% of the next $500,000
- 15% of anything above $600,000

Let's say you have a case that settles out of court for $300,000. Attorneys' and experts expenses totaled $34,308.67. The attorney, under the statute, would be paid the expenses of $34,308.67 plus 40% of the first $50,000 ($20,000) plus 33.3% of the next $50,000 ($16,666.66) plus 25% of $165,691.32 ($41,422.83) for a total of $102,398.16. The plaintiff would receive $187,601.84.

A medical malpractice plaintiff's attorney will frequently be asked to take on a case in which they statistically have only a 20% to 25% chance of winning the case, whether it is arbitrated or tried.

From Winer's experience as a plaintiff's attorney, he or she will have to pay out an average of $75,000 in costs that are deducted from potential attorney's fees, leaving the attorney a fee of about $55,000 with an award (at the cap limit) of $250,000. The plaintiff will only recover $120,000, sometimes for a life-ending or life-destroying injury in such a scenario after deducting expenses and attorney fees. This example does not consider future medical expenses and out of pocket medical expenses to date.

It is nothing for a plaintiff's attorney to incur $75,000 in fees to mount a case. These fees are paid out of the settlement money, if any, otherwise the plaintiff pays them.

If the attorney firm only earns $55,000 in fees for prevailing in or out of court, and 750 hours of attorney time are required (which is quite common), the attorney works for $73 per hour for a 75% chance of losing.

As you can see, the numbers aren't good for the plaintiff or the plaintiff's attorney.

The system is slanted against any injured party who pursues a case.

Where will the attorneys' expense money come from?

It is common for contracts (with the plaintiff) for medical malpractice contingent attorneys' fees to indicate that the attorney or law firm handling your case may ask you to finance the cost of your case. In other words, the case will not proceed unless you pay the attorney some money.

In practice, most attorneys who take medical malpractice cases cannot "float" the cost of experts up front in going to trial or arbitration. In other kinds of injury cases, no recovery, no fee for the lawyer's time. In medical malpractice cases, experts do not work for free or work on "the come."

This discourages the pursuit of medical malpractice lawsuits in California. It also encourages a settlement of less than the value of the case because the plaintiff does not have the money to get the damages that the plaintiff thinks that he/she deserves.

Plaintiffs' attorneys have an incentive to settle cases since any legal expenses are deducted from settlement monies before attorneys' fees are calculated. Fewer expenses mean more money for a plaintiff's attorney.

Why do you need an attorney?

Without question, if you have a medical malpractice case in California, you need an attorney. Specifically, you need a medical malpractice attorney.

Medical malpractice law is a highly technical field of law. Such cases are vigorously defended by well-funded defense firms who represent medical malpractice insurance companies.

Due to the technical skills necessary to prosecute such a case, the possibility exists that an inexperienced or non-specialized lawyer might not be sufficiently conversant with med mal law or medical procedures and is at a disadvantage in such a scenario.

In general, the higher the amount of the monetary settlement, the more scrutiny the Medical Board of California will give to a particular case. Defendants do not want to be put under a microscope. This convinces many defendants to settle out-of-court.

The drama of a medical malpractice case acts against plaintiffs and to the benefit of the defendant medical malpractice insurance carriers. Being a plaintiff in a medical malpractice case is stressful. Without belaboring the point, extreme stress over a long period of time can create physical and emotional problems.

When is *informed consent* necessary?

Except in emergency situations, a healthcare provider must obtain consent from a patient.

It is a healthcare provider's duty to provide *informed consent* with enough knowledge for a patient in order for the patient to make an informed choice. The healthcare provider should give the patient sufficient pertinent information and material to make that decision.

The healthcare provider must explain the procedure and the risk of the procedure in a way that a layperson can understand it. The healthcare provider must give the patient an opportunity to weigh the risks.

The burden of proof requires a connection between the failure to inform and the injury.

For a plaintiff to prevail in an informed consent case, the patient must establish a causal relationship between the healthcare provider's failure to inform and the injury to the plaintiff. In these types of cases, it must be established that had the revelation been made, consent to treatment would not have been given.

Patients must be informed not only of the risks inherent in the procedure in question, but also the risks of not choosing the treatment or procedure.

When is an *informed consent* not necessary?

Any healthcare provider can defend the failure to adequately inform the patient by asserting:

- An emergency situation
- The patient was unconscious and the healthcare provider believed the procedure needed to be performed immediately and there was insufficient time to tell the patient.
- The patient was not capable of giving consent (e.g., a minor) and the healthcare provider reasonably believed the procedure was immediately necessary and that there was insufficient time to obtain consent from a parent.
- Additional surgery is necessary due to conditions arising during an operation which endangers the patient's health or life.
- When there is no reason why the patient would not have requested the treatment, even if the condition is not life-threatening, if the additional treatment is a requirement because of a complication in the course of the procedure.
- The patient specifically asked not to be informed.
- Where a doctor can offer proof that the disclosure would have seriously upset patient to the degree that the patient would not have been able to objectively weigh the risks of refusing to undergo the recommended treatment.

What constitutes *a substantial factors* causation standard?

      A plaintiff does not have to prove that the defendant's negligence was the one and only cause of a plaintiff's injury but that it was a *substantial factor* in causing the injury. Still, almost by definition, the plaintiff suffered from "an injury" or medical condition before the treatment in question in a medical malpractice case.

      The defense will frequently make one of the following claims to support its position:

- The injury claimed is a natural progression of the condition which the plaintiff sought treatment for from the defendant, and the defendant did not further aggravate that condition by his or her negligence.
- Although the healthcare provider violated the standard of care, the plaintiff's condition was incurable; therefore, negligence during treatment did not cause any injury. (This is a frequent defense in failure to diagnose cancer cases.)
- Even if the defendant was negligent in diagnosing a condition sooner, an earlier diagnosis would not have changed the outcome in a particular case.
- The patient's injury that is claimed has nothing at all to do with the defendant's treatment but developed independently of whatever the defendant did wrong.
- Even when the defendant violated the standard of care by a failure to use appropriate diagnostic techniques, the injured plaintiff's condition would not have been discovered even if proper diagnostic techniques were utilized.

Did you know that *causation defenses* are sometimes used to confuse jurors?

      In California, 80% of medical malpractice cases that go to trial are won by defendant doctors thanks in large part to effective *causation defenses*.

Many variations of the causation "defenses" exist. They are limited only by the extent of the imagination of the healthcare provider, his trial experts and his defense attorney. These causation defenses, including the valid ones, are frequently utilized by the defense to confuse trial jurors and to provide the jurors with a reason to find for the defense, even when there has been clear negligence. Never mind "the truth."

Why does a plaintiff need *expert testimony* in a medical malpractice case?

Expert testimony is generally required to prove a violation of the standard of care in a medical malpractice case. When used, expert testimony is required to establish customary medical practices in the community and what the appropriate practice would be under the circumstances presented in a particular case.

Expert testimony is also required to prove a causal link between the plaintiff's injury and the healthcare provider's negligence.

When is expert testimony *not* needed?

The single exception to the requirement of expert testimony is the rare case in which the negligence of a healthcare provider can be demonstrated by facts through common knowledge.

These cases are extremely rare. If the defense secures an expert who testifies that the obvious negligence was within the standard of care, and it was, the plaintiff will probably lose.

What is significant about a *battle of the experts* in a medical malpractice case?

Medical malpractice cases frequently come down to a *battle of experts*. A plaintiff's case can be helped if the jurors, either by common sense or life experience, realize that defendant healthcare provider should have done something differently.

How expensive are medical malpractice experts?

Expert witnesses in medical malpractice cases are very expensive. Many charge well over $500 per hour to review records and give sworn testimony. It is common that thousands of pages of relevant medical records and thousands and thousands more pages of deposition (sworn out-of-court testimony) must be reviewed by the experts. A single expert in a medical malpractice case may charge $25,000 to $50,000 by the end of the trial. It can cost over $5,000 just for a plaintiff to learn whether or not there is a valid case.

More than one expert witness is often required to prove a medical malpractice case. Sometimes there will be more than one specialist who committed malpractice. There may be a hospital involved and a family doctor who is alleged to have been negligent. In such cases, the plaintiff may have to retain a hospital expert, a general practitioner and more than one specialist as experts. Furthermore, it may be necessary to retain yet another expert on the causation issue in order to prove that the malpractice caused the injury.

The defense almost always hires many experts, thus putting the plaintiff at a disadvantage if he or she does not match the defense expert for expert.

What is the *Conspiracy of Silence*?

Plaintiffs can encounter a great deal of difficulty finding doctors willing to testify in medical malpractice cases against defendant doctors. Many doctors feel uncomfortable testifying against a colleague, even if it is somebody they do not know.

With damage limitations placed on plaintiffs, and fee limitations on their attorneys in medical malpractice cases, it is unwise to bring a medical malpractice case unless there is fairly clear liability, causation and substantial damages.

Some medical malpractice cases involve birth and obstetricians. Why are obstetrical malpractice insurance premiums so high?

Obstetrical malpractice cases frequently require experts from several specialties and are almost always very complicated which makes them expensive to pursue.

Awards in the tens of millions of dollars over their lifetime to injured plaintiffs in obstetrical malpractice cases have occurred and will occur in the future.

The most challenging medical malpractice cases usually involve the very serious neurological and other systemic problems that a baby can develop during the pregnancy and birth processes. Most commonly, these involve improper monitoring during the pregnancy, birth and immediate post-birth periods. When that is the case, a baby can develop cerebral palsy and other extraordinarily serious illnesses and disabilities which can severely shorten the newborn's life expectancy and/or require a lifetime of attendant care.

What about altered medical records?

When a plaintiff can establish that the chart was altered or deceitfully filled out, based on testimony of nurses or evidence that a doctor was not called when the chart says he or she was called, this will greatly increase the likelihood that the plaintiff will prevail — not only in a medical malpractice case, but also in a fraud case.

What about medical malpractice cases involving surgeries?

The nature of a medical malpractice case will differ depending upon the particular surgery in question. Most cases will have several common themes.

Regarding elective surgeries, a potential lawsuit has to determine whether the surgery should have been performed at all.

The claimed malpractice in a surgery case may be that there were not enough indications, based on the patient's signs and symptoms, to perform the surgery rather than some less risky or invasive treatment. Two examples of this kind of case are when an obstetrician performs a hysterectomy which was not necessary; or a doctor performs open heart surgery when a less radical form of treatment, such as performing an angioplasty, would have been indicated.

In some cases, particularly those involving cosmetic surgery, the malpractice claim could be that the physician performed the surgery simply to make money.

Why is a pre-surgery workup necessary?

Almost all hospitals require a patient to be examined by an Internal Medicine member of the staff before the surgery. An alternative is to have the patient's own doctor submit a written report on the patient's general health, based on a recent pre-surgical examination.

In addition, the anesthesiologist has to perform some type of examination and question the patient before surgery.

Sometimes appropriate information is not communicated between the doctors or they fail to perform the appropriate tests, given the patient's signs and symptoms, to diagnose and recognize a problem which should result in the surgery being postponed or canceled.

What constitutes a surgical error?

Medical malpractice cases that focus on surgical mistakes can involve investigations of a large multitude of problems ranging from slipped scalpels, nerves that were unnecessarily cut, improperly administered and monitored anesthesia, infections caused by unsterile tools and any number of other errors.

These cases are difficult to prove at times because the surgeon and anesthesiologist will make notes indicating proper protocol was followed and a surgeon will dictate an operation report which conforms to the standard of care.

Sometimes the malpractice is not discovered until the patient requires another surgery and the second surgeon discovers what was done improperly in the earlier surgery. Other times, the mistake will be discovered as a result of the patient's poor result. In some cases, the mistake will never be discovered or proven, despite a bad surgical outcome.

What are common defenses to surgical malpractice cases?

Surgeons will defend such cases by claiming that the poor result was a known risk of the surgery and, frequently, the patient will have signed an informed consent sheet indicating he or she knew the risk.

However, this does not preclude a claim for malpractice if the surgeon did not conform to the standard of care in performing the surgery and the poor result was caused by a violation of the standard of care.

In some cases, surgeons may claim that they are not an insurer of the success of an operation as not every surgery is successful. The plaintiff will lose unless he or she can establish a violation of the standard of care and that the poor result was caused by the violation of the standard of care and was not a failure which can be reasonably anticipated in this type of operation.

Generally speaking, it is very difficult to prevail in a medical malpractice surgery case if the only claim is that the surgery did not work. The surgeon being sued simply asserts that bad results occur a given percentage of the time with even the best surgeons performing the surgery by showing statistics.

The better surgery malpractice cases from the plaintiff's point of view involve serious complications that occur during the surgery, which would not have occurred unless the surgeon or anesthesiologist violated the standard of care. For example, a case in which the patient becomes brain-damaged as a result of the anesthesiologist's failure to monitor oxygen flow to the brain or a case in which the surgeon fails to monitor the patient's loss of blood and the patient dies. These cases not only end up with a bad result, but there is also **proof of negligence.**

What are some areas of concern in *failure to prescribe the appropriate medicine* cases?

- Failure to prescribe the **appropriate dosage** of medicine

- Failure to prescribe the medicine for **an appropriate period of time**
- **Misprescription of medicine** (i.e., the wrong medicine)
- **Failure to properly monitor blood levels**, when indicated, for certain medicines
- **Acting beyond expertise** in treating a patient
- **Failure to adequately instruct the patient** as to home care or when to return to the office if problems result
- **Failure to seek appropriate consultation** with another doctor or specialist
- **Failure to follow a patient or arrange for appropriate follow-up** when a patient is hospitalized
- **Failure to adequately respond to emergencies**

The importance in all malpractice cases is proving a standard of care violation and causation.

What about The MICRA and *wrongful death cases*?

If a person dies as a result of medical malpractice, and leaves many heirs behind, such as a spouse and children, the total amount of money that the entire family can recover for non-economic damages is $250,000. That's all that is allowed under the law. A plaintiff can sue for incurred medical costs.

In a case in which a number of doctors and a hospital are proven to cause a plaintiff's death the plaintiff's total recovery against all the doctors and the hospital is a single $250,000 non-economic damages award.

Did you know that if the plaintiff lives to receive an award and later dies as a result of the malpractice his heirs can collect again?

When a plaintiff receives a serious injury, he or she can collect up to a $250,000 non-economic damage cap. If a patient later dies from the malpractice injuries, the heirs, all together, can collect up to $250,000.

It should be noted that the $250,000 damage cap is, in fact, only a "cap"; frequently jurors or arbitrators award less than $250,000 in non-economic damages in a medical malpractice case.

How do periodic payments for future damage awards work under The MICRA?

Under The MICRA, future damage awards of $50,000 or more against medical malpractice defendants can be paid over time by the healthcare provider or their insurance company.

A person is entitled to a payment of his award for future income loss, medical expenses, attendant care needs or general damages at the time the award is made by a judge, jury or arbitrator in all personal injury cases *other than* medical malpractice cases.

Thus, plaintiff's money that should be due them at the time of their award will be worth less when they are received than they were at the time of the award because of inflation. This punishes a plaintiff.

Obviously, $50,000 today is worth far less than $50,000 was thirty years ago. The same will be true for a $50,000 payment thirty years into the future. There is no mechanism to correct this. Obviously, there should be.

This makes it very difficult for the plaintiff to receive emotional closure in very emotional cases. Whenever the periodic payments are made, the plaintiff will have yet another reminder of the ordeal. In fact, insurance companies usually do not want to make payments over time any more than a plaintiff wants to receive them. So they will pay it all at one time.

As far as periodic payments that are allowed under The MICRA are concerned, plaintiff's attorneys would rather see all the money upfront at the time of a settlement. So would plaintiffs.

Can claims for *loss of consortium* be filed?

A plaintiff's spouse can also sue and recover damages for *loss of consortium*. A spouse is allowed to recover damages for the loss of society, comfort and care that result from the injured spouse's unavailability due to their injury. In order to recover these damages, a spouse must be named as a party to the lawsuit and must have been married to the plaintiff at the time of the injury.

There are advantages and disadvantages to filing a loss of consortium claim that should be discussed with an attorney before filing.

What are the rules of The MICRA concerning minors?

A different statute of limitations for minors' medical malpractice negligence cases exists than for any other kind of case. Usually a minor has until he or she turns nineteen to bring a lawsuit. A case by a minor for medical negligence injuries must be brought within three years from the date of the alleged wrongful act. If the minor is under the age of six when the wrongful act occurred, the medical malpractice action must be filed within three years or prior to the minor's eighth birthday, whichever period is longer. (Minors are bound by the six-month claim statute in cases against public entities.)

The one-year/three-year statute of limitations **only** applies to medical negligence causes of action.

In some medical malpractice cases, particularly cases involving sexual abuse by a physician, a plaintiff will plead a number of causes of action in addition to medical negligence. These causes of action are not affected by the one-year/three-year statute, and most of them begin to run within one or two years from the date of the discovery of harm with no three-year outside limitation.

What are the effects on The MICRA limitations on the feasibility of bringing a medical malpractice action and the possibility of a fair settlement?

Remember, The MICRA limitations were intended to limits victims' rights.

The MICRA laws were written to have the effect of severely limiting the number of medical malpractice actions that are brought in California and the number of attorneys who are willing to handle medical malpractice cases.

The healthcare industry pushed through The MICRA limitations via an extraordinarily intensive lobbying effort. That effort to retain The MICRA limitations continues.

The MICRA limitations, added to the difficulties in prevailing in a medical malpractice case in general, have created a situation in which many righteous medical malpractice victims are either unable to find attorneys to handle their case or are grossly undercompensated when they do bring a case and win.

The $250,000 non-economic damage cap unjustly punishes the most severely injured and disabled malpractice victims and victims of disfigurement. On the other hand, if a person only suffered a mild to moderate injury as a result of the malpractice, their damages might not even reach the $250,000 cap and they will be fully compensated unless periodic payments are used.

A person whose life was totally wrecked by malpractice, such as a non-working spouse who becomes a quadriplegic as the result of malpractice, will only receive maybe one hundredth of fair compensation, since a jury will be likely to award as much as $20,000,000 for general damages in that type of case. The judge in such a case, bound by the statute, will reduce the non-economic damages reward to only $250,000.

How can medical malpractice insurance companies abuse the $250,000 general damage cap?

Healthcare providers and their insurance companies abuse the $250,000 general damage cap. In clear liability catastrophic injury cases, they have nothing to lose by offering, let's say, $200,000 for non-economic damages. This forces the plaintiff to trial where the plaintiff may have to spend an additional $50,000 or more to increase the award by $50,000.

Why is there is an enormous disincentive for attorneys to handle malpractice cases and what are the financial risks of a malpractice case?

First, start with the idea that only 25% of medical malpractice cases that are tried or arbitrated result in a victory for the patient. Add to that the possibility that the medical malpractice case will easily cost (excluding attorneys fees) $50,000 or more to try or arbitrate. Then throw in a $250,000 cap on non-economic damages and you can see how the disincentive comes into play.

For most malpractice victims, the $250,000 represents the total amount of money that can be awarded because they have health insurance to pay medical bills and many do not have any significant wage loss claims. You can see why an attorney would be hesitant to bring a medical malpractice case when there is so little upside and so much downside.

This doesn't even consider that the attorney's fees will be limited to less than two-thirds of what an attorney could earn on other, often easier, personal injury cases.

Since most medical malpractice cases do not settle early, even if there is a settlement before trial, case costs will normally be over $25,000 and as high as $100,000 or more.

Under The MICRA, the attorney is only entitled to his or her percentage after the case costs are deducted from the client's verdict or settlement.

This is not a lucrative situation for an attorney nor a plaintiff.

Why is there a unlikely prospect of an early settlement?

A defendant doctor has the absolute right to refuse consent to settle a case against him or her. Mix this with the fact that medical malpractice cases are usually intensely litigated with a large number of depositions and attorney time spent on a case. Even if an insurance company wants to settle a case, or settle a case early, it will sometimes not be allowed to do so. Doctors do not want their reputations hurt, and they will push the case through to a trial with nothing financially to lose if they feel they can prevail. Why? Because the insurance company will pay for any verdict rendered against them.

Why do medical malpractice victims have so much trouble finding attorneys?

The situation mentioned above is obviously worse where there is not a major injury and a verdict or settlement might be substantially less than $250,000.

This is why righteous medical malpractice victims sometimes have to contact dozens of attorneys before they either give up or can find an attorney to handle their case. In the real world, many will not be able to find an attorney at all.

Will good attorneys still handle malpractice cases after careful screening?

This is not all doom and gloom. There are very good attorneys will still handle medical malpractice cases.

Unfortunately, they may only accept cases in which there is some way around The MICRA limitations — such as intentional tort (involves intentional acts), sexual abuse or elder abuse — or the liability in the case is extraordinarily clear, and the potential damage recovery is more than $250,000. The point of view of the plaintiff's attorney is to assess the chances of winning at the very beginning of the case to see if the case will fall within the 25% of cases that can win.

If the plaintiff presents that type of case, the chances are greater that the case will settle without a trial or arbitration, and if it has to be tried or arbitrated, the plaintiff has at least a 50-50 chance of winning. Thus, medical malpractice cases are carefully screened by good attorneys.

Can attorneys without experience obtain good results in malpractice cases?

Plaintiffs sometimes end up being represented by attorneys without substantial medical malpractice experience. This may happen because the plaintiffs do not know any better or an attorney without medical malpractice experience may not recognize the expenses and risks outlined above and wrongfully believe that a medical malpractice case can be settled easily without the outlay of great expense and time. A number of these attorneys will drop a case after it has been filed when they understand what they have gotten themselves into. The plaintiff is left to try to find another attorney. This is an unfortunately common set of circumstances.

Why is a *review of medical records* so important?

The primary investigation of a medical malpractice case centers on the receipt and review of medical records. Most medical malpractice cases rise or fall on the basis of what is included in the medical records by those who provided treatment and care before the injury occurred or before it was discovered.

Most medical records are extraordinarily difficult to read. They must be read by someone who is able to decipher the notes, even if that ends up involving the deposition of the person who wrote the notes if the notes appear at all critical.

Medical records, particularly records of hospitals, are usually not in any chronological order. To be able to correctly analyze a medical malpractice case, someone reviewing all these notes must put them in chronological order to show what happened.

It is only by putting all the records into chronological order that someone reviewing them will be able to truly understand what happened to the plaintiff. This work enables the reviewer to find inconsistencies in the notes, such as when a doctor notes a normal blood pressure on an examination at the exact same time that a nurse notes a grossly abnormal blood pressure.

The notes must be investigated with the eye toward the possibility of missing or altered notes. Having the notes in chronological order is an aid to finding notes that should be present but are missing and inconsistent notes which may lead an investigator to believe the notes have been altered.

If the supposition is that the records may have been altered, the plaintiff may want to consider hiring a handwriting analysis expert to review the records. Additionally, it is often fruitful to review records from other patients made at a similar time.

What about *statements and testimony of nurses and office staff*?

It is common for the nurses at a hospital to rally around a hospital to defend a medical malpractice claim under investigation. The same is true of nurses and employees of doctors in cases involving outpatient chart entries.

In a situation in which a number of nurses have to keep their stories straight in order for a hospital to prevail, a plaintiff attorney may be able to turn up inconsistencies between the stories of the various nurses. This will help to create evidence of malpractice from their individual depositions.

Why are medical malpractice cases difficult to settle?

According to Winer, in California, almost all doctors are insured by "doctor-owned" insurance companies that are committed to spending whatever it takes to win a malpractice case rather than pay a settlement to a plaintiff. Further complicating the settlment process, doctors are allowed to refuse consent to settle a medical malpractice case and frequently do refuse consent even if their attorney or insurance carrier urges otherwise.

In the hope of obtaining a significant out-of-court settlement, a plaintiff's attorney makes sure that the doctor and insurance company understand the risk of not settling and proceeding to trial. In other words, a trial has to be perceived as having a greater potential award than settling out of court.

How is this accomplished?

It is better to be open and upfront starting at the beginning of the case as to what the plaintiff's experts will testify to under oath and the facts and evidence which the plaintiff believes will result in a verdict for the plaintiff. If not taking this approach, considerable time and sometimes an obscene amount of money will be spent on preparing and trying the case — which, statistics show, the plaintiff has only a 25% chance at best of winning.

The downside of this approach is that it gives the defense more information than it would usually have to prepare a defense to defeat the claim.

What about arbitration cases?

Plaintiffs prevail in 40% of all arbitrations supposedly because there is no jury in place which might be sympathetic to a doctor or doctors.

Many times, HMOs, especially Kaiser, only use arbitration to settle medical malpractice cases.

Sometimes a plaintiff will have to pay part of the arbitration cost.

The real protection that HMOs seek in arbitration is that an arbitrator is far less likely to make a large punitive damage award against the HMO than would be an angry jury. Further, jurors would be much more likely to rule for the plaintiff in malpractice cases against HMOs than cases against individual doctors.

The major complaint from plaintiffs in Kaiser Arbitrations is that it is difficult to find a "neutral" arbitrator according to Winer's guide. Kaiser keeps a list of all arbitrators in its cases and then it carefully monitors the award given by each arbitrator in each case. If you read between the lines, you can see why this is problematic for plaintiffs when Kaiser selects from arbitrators the3y have used previously.

Again, this is an abridged look at Winer's guide.

*****

265

The preceding is why you should have your head examined before you file a medical malpractice lawsuit in California.

*****

In the next chapter, we will look at efforts to reform The MICRA and med mal legislation in general, as well as the push-back to prevent such reforms. As a weary and outraged survivor of the medical malpractice system in California, I was curious and anxious to find ideas for improving the situation in my state and nationwide.

Chapter 17—Thoughts about Medical Malpractice Reform

As it stands today, California's MICRA statute is badly out of date. Some federally elected officials have discussed the possibility of California MICRA-type legislation on a national basis.

The reforms I've written about in this book can be applied to any California MICRA-based system such as the Texas and Nevada laws. They are also applicable to states who may want to enact a California MICRA-type statute.

The ongoing debate about MICRA is highly contentious. So are many of the California cases settled under MICRA provisions. On the one side, we have physicians and medical malpractice carriers who say the current caps are still necessary. On the other side, there are the California medical malpractice plaintiffs' attorneys, reformists and patient safety advocates, who are asking for raising the cap on non-economic damages and other reforms. The Internet contains thousands of postings — both pro reform and con.

My first thought about MICRA reform had to do with an increased cap on non-economic damages in med mal cases. It is too low at $250,000. This was my thinking prior to doing any research. As I did the research, I saw that there is more to the story — and that, at the same time, the caps were an essential piece of it. This chapter shares my exploration of The MICRA controversy.

*****

On June 13, 1993, then former California Governor Edmund Gerald "Jerry" Brown, Jr. made a statement about The MICRA. Excerpts from that statement follow.

The then former Governor talked about the medical malpractice insurance "crisis" that had led to the development and passage of The MICRA because it seemed critical to the healthcare system in the State in 1975.

Continuing on, he said, "We have learned a lot about MICRA and the insurance industry in the seventeen years since MICRA was enacted. We have even witnessed yet another insurance industry crisis, and found that insurance company avarice, not utilization of the legal system by injured consumers, was responsible for excessive premiums. Saddest of all, MICRA has revealed itself to have an arbitrary and cruel effect upon victims of malpractice. It has not lowered healthcare costs, only enriched insurers and placed negligent or incompetent physicians outside the reach of judicial accountability. For these reasons, MICRA cannot and should not be a model for national legislation."[xvii]

According to attorney and political blogger Brian Leubitz, "The ($250,000 MICRA) cap doesn't change (medical malpractice) insurance rates, but does take away the accountability that the tort system provides. The limit is hurting victims of malpractice and their families."[xviii]

A Search for Numbers

On April 8, 2013, I sent an email to California's Department of Public Health asking them how many patients die in the State each year due to preventable medical errors.

In their response, they referred me to the State's Medical Board.

Later that same day, I sent an email to the Medical Board of California asking them the same question.

In a return email, Chris Valine wrote, "The Medical Board does not track the number of patients who die each year in California due to medical malpractice."

That struck me as very odd since the Medical Board of California receives complaints about medical malpractice, some of which involve deceased patients. If not them, then who has the statistics?

A Look at the Patient Advocacy Groups

In my research, I discovered that many patient advocacy organizations in California are actively lobbying the State Legislature regarding medical malpractice reforms and patient safety reforms. With limited funding, they are attempting to improve patient safety and improve malpractice reporting.

On their websites, some of them post horrific stories of medical malpractice negligence and some name doctors and healthcare facilities who have been sued over and over again for the same type of errors.

How do healthcare providers get away with it?

Here's one way… If a healthcare provider settles a case for $30,000 or less, no report of the malpractice is made to the Medical Board of California as part of any settlement.

James W. Hurt, Jr. of Hurt, Stolz and Cromwell, LLC blogged on April 17, 2013 that according to the Centers for Disease Control and Prevention (CDC) that as a result of analyzing court documents in the U.S. that nearly 100,000 wrongful death claims for medical malpractice are filed against healthcare providers each year. [xix]

I believe that the number of deaths attributable to medical malpractice is really higher than what the CDC reported since it seems likely to me all of these types of incidents do not result in lawsuits.

ASAP (Alliance for Safety Awareness for Patients — PatientSafetyASAP.org), founded by med mal survivor Alicia Cole, is one of the activist organizations. The main thrust of the group is to eliminate hospital-acquired infections and promote transparency in reporting errant physicians.

Another group had the answer to my original question about the numbers and more info on infections. According to a March 2010 document titled "Preventable Harm," **Consumers Union SafePatientProject.org says, "An estimated 240,000 California patients develop infections in hospitals each year, resulting in an estimated 13,500 deaths per year at a cost of $3.1 billion per year… Medical errors kill as many as 10,000 Californians each year and injure 140,000 patients."**[xx]

Consumers Union runs The Safe Patient Project campaign. SPP's website (SafePatientProject.org) posts peoples' heartfelt stories about medical malpractice incidents. They offer the stories as a backdrop for advocating change for patient care reform, as well as medical malpractice reporting of physicians and healthcare providers.

A very knowledgeable, unnamed source regarding lobbying for patients' rights in California told me that, "For those who aren't aware of it, the Medical Board of California was established to protect medical patients but it is common knowledge that, in practice, it protects many bad doctors at the expense of injured patients.

Apparently the Medical Board of California must re-apply for renewal every ten years or so. Prior to the renewal, the Sunset Hearings for the Medical Board of California are held. In theory, the Sunset Hearing is held to determine whether or not the Medical Board of California should continue.

On March 11, 2013, the day after the most recent Sunset Hearing in Sacramento, many people from the Safe Patient Project lobbied in the State Capitol that the Board is not transparent and that there is an unwillingness to investigate or discipline some physicians who are responsible for patient deaths. Med mal insurers know, local medical boards know, some hospitals know, but not the general public. Aides to some elected officials said that many State Assembly members get too much campaign money from the California Medical Association to ever abolish the Medical Board of California — let alone reprimand it. It is horrible that there is such insidious, unbelievable corruption in every layer of the medical culture and politics in California."

Another group in California and elsewhere that advocates for better/safer patient care is **Consumer Watchdog (ConsumerWatchdog.org)**.

Jamie Court of Consumer Watchdog recently said that the Medical Board of California is somewhat akin to a racket allowing protection for the State's worst doctors, the ones who continue to dole out substandard care to different patients repeatedly thus injuring them.

What Are the Patient Advocates Calling For?

During a two-day session lobbying in the State Capitol with aides to California legislators in March 2013, some members of **The Safe Patient Project** advocated that:

- All med mal lawsuit awards exceeding $30,000 should be posted on the Medical Board of California website.
- Physicians receiving the Medical Board of California disciplinary probation must notify their patients of the action.
- The need for having faster reporting of complaints against healthcare providers is necessary.
- Reporting of all cases of medical malpractice and having posted notices in the offices of healthcare providers and institutions offering healthcare about where complaints can be filed.[xxi]

Alicia Cole, Founder of the Alliance for Safety Awareness for Patients (ASAP), shared that the original surgeon who operated on her and injured her due to medical malpractice shows *no* medical malpractice judgments against him. This is despite the fact that he has had six cases against him for medical malpractice, two of which settled for over $30,000.

Ms. Cole has called for the Sunset Review Board to review the laws about reporting preventable medical errors on the website of the Medical Board of California. This was proposed by the Medical Board staff very recently but was not enacted by the physician-controlled Board.[xxii]

Patient care advocate groups want transparency for medical errors by all healthcare providers and real enforcement against substandard caregivers by the Medical Board of California. At present, these groups do not feel that either area is anywhere close to what it needs to be.

LA Times Coverage Shines Light on the Issues

One of the most powerful voices for changes to improve patient safety in California has been *The Los Angeles Times.*

On April 7, 2011, an article by *Times* reporter Eryn Brown appeared titled "Medical Errors in Hospitals Go Undetected, Study Suggests." Brown noted that researchers from the think tank, Institute for Health Improvement, reported that preventable medical errors might be ten times greater than previously measured in a 1999 landmark study. The earlier Institute of Medicine study reported that medical errors in U.S. hospitals are linked to "tens of thousands" of deaths each year.[xxiii]

On February 8, 2012, there was a piece from *Times* reporter Karen Kaplan called "Many Doctors Hide the Truth about Medical Errors, Study Finds." The story involved a nationwide survey of roughly 1,800 physicians by the Mongan Institute for Health Policy at Massachusetts General Hospital in Boston. Thirty-four percent of the physicians surveyed "did not completely agree" that "all significant medical errors" should be made known to patients. In the previous year, 20% of those surveyed had not disclosed information about their medical mistakes. Interestingly, general surgeons and pediatricians were the medical specialists most likely to say that serious medical errors should be made known to patients. Cardiologists and psychiatrists disagreed with that idea most often.[xxiv]

On June 6, 2012, *Times* reporter Chad Terhune wrote an article titled "41% of California Hospitals Graded C or Lower on Patient Safety." The piece covered a new grading program of hospital performance in the area of patient safety. The purpose of the grading by the Leapfrog Group was to push hospitals to do more to prevent thousands of mistakes and deaths. A Leapfrog spokesperson said the grading system was inspired by effectiveness of the alphabetical restaurant grading program. All hospitals receiving a potential grading of lower than C by Leapfrog had until November to make improvements before a grade of D or F would be assigned to them. Ronald Reagan UCLA Medical Center was among that group. **Northridge Hospital Medical Center** received a grade below C. [xxv]

On November 11, 2012, an investigative article by *Times* reporters Scott Glover and Lisa Girion was featured titled "Legal Drugs, Deadly Outcomes." Their reportage, which included researching coroners' records, detailed how a "small number" of physicians could be tied to a "disproportionate number of prescriptions" believed to have caused or contributed to fatal overdoses. The tagline of the piece read, "Prescription overdoses kill more people than heroin and cocaine."[xxvi]

I feel that this article may have helped to motivate families of the deceased prescription drug overdose patients to testify before the Sunset Review in March 2013 about the lack of scrutiny and enforcement against the doctors in question.

On November 28, 2012, *Times* writer Chad Terhune authored an article titled "UCLA Medical Center Gets Failing Grade on Patient Safety." Terhune noted that the Ronald Reagan UCLA Medical Center, a prestigious Los Angeles hospital, was one of only twenty-five hospitals out of the 2,652 studied nationwide to receive a failing grade. The article was covering an update to Leapfrog's first-time-ever grading report issued in June.

Officials at the UCLA Medical Center disputed the finding that they deserved an F for poor performance on several levels related to "preventing medical errors, patient infections and deaths."

The California Hospital Association thought highly of Leapfrog for its work. [xxvii]

(For the latest hospital scores from Leapfrog, go to www.hospitalsafetyscore.org.)

On March 13, 2013, an article by The Partnership at Drugfree.org (Join Together Staff) appeared titled "California Legislators: Use Database to Find Doctors who Overprescribe Painkillers." In it, the writers printed remarks from Assemblyman Richard Gordon as saying, in essence, that the State Legislature needed to become proactive in looking for patterns of overprescribing some potentially harmful prescription drugs since doctors receive huge amounts of money for prescribing them. [xxviii]

Opponents said that using such tactic might cause doctors not to prescribe painkillers for legitimate purposes.

*****

As you can see, the issue of medical malpractice as it relates to patient safety is being highly scrutinized by consumers, the press, and some state officials. Medical malpractice insurers, their lobbyists, and some physician groups want to keep The MICRA as it is.

*****

Pressure on California's Medical Board

On April 1, 2013, California State Senator Curren D. Price, Jr. and California Assemblyman Richard Gordon notified Medical Board of California President Sharon Levine, MD, via a letter[xxix] that unless the Board made firm commitments and significant progress in the areas of: **Enforcement Program Shortfalls, Vertical Enforcement Prosecution, Adoption of Uniform Substance Abuse Standards** (against medical practitioners), **Consumer Protection Enforcement Provisions, Oversight of Surgical Clinics, Stipulated Settlements Below the Disciplinary Guidelines, and Use of Interim Suspension Authority** that the Sunset Extensions for the Medical Board of California and the Board's Executive Director will be removed from the Sunset legislation.

In short, Ms. Levine was told that the Board needed to clean up its act or it would be history.

Assemblyman Gordon and Senator Price wrote to Ms. Levine that Californians needed a proactive Medical Board that considered patients first and doctors' interests secondarily.

Legislators and the Governor are all ears

On July 1, 2013, Governor Jerry Brown, State Senate President Pro-tempore Darrell Steinberg and Assembly Speaker John A . Perez listened to pleas from Californians represented by **38 Is Too Late**, co-chaired by Bob Pack, to reform or eliminate two key provisions of The MICRA: The $250,000 cap on non-economic damages; the wrongful death cap of $250,000. [xxx] www.38istoolate.org

Senator Steinberg said in early May 2013 that he would hold hearings on The MICRA cap for victims' recovery. He spoke on the sidewalk of the State Capitol to injured patients and their families. [xxxi]

274

Med Mal Reforms Suggested by Dr. Marty Makary

Just so you don't think that all physicians want to hide the truth about the realities of medical malpractice, I'm going to cover suggestions for med mal reform offered by Marty Makary, MD. Dr. Makary is a surgeon at Johns Hopkins University, the developer of a safety checklist for surgical procedures used by the World Health Organization, and the author of *Unaccountable: What Hospitals Won't Tell You and How Transparency Can Revolutionize Health Care*. In a December 8, 2012 interview about this title on C-SPAN's *BookTV*, Dr. Makary had plenty to say about accountability and transparency in healthcare.

He noted that physicians as a whole are under great pressure with declining Medicare payments, rising overhead, and an increase in medical malpractice insurance premiums. On top of that, he referred to a recent study conducted by the Mayo Clinic which showed that 46% of all U.S. doctors suffer some degree of burnout.

As a 3rd year medical student, Dr. Makary quit medical school as he was frustrated with the lack of transparency and accountability for medical mistakes among colleagues and instructors at his medical school. At that point, he switched to a doctoral program in public health where he was introduced to the idea of accountability and transparency regarding patient care. The doctor noted that that field is generating a lot of interest among some doctors, healthcare administrators, hospital executives and healthcare organizations. He said that it is a rapidly growing trend. He noted that he found that people in New York City are more likely to review restaurants online than hospitals. He said that medical errors are the third leading cause of death in the United States.[xxxii]

In a *Wall Street Journal* article, Dr. Makary noted that from his own experience, once a doctor is trained and providing medical care, the doctor is bound by an unwritten/unspoken rule to overlook any medical mistakes made by other doctors. According to Makary, this is wrong because it does nothing to aid in the reduction of medical mistakes. He goes further saying that by reporting wrongdoing, the reporting doctor is ostracized and that results in a severe economic impact against the doctor. In his mind, such a system discourages reporting on colleagues about their medical errors.

Dr. Makary said that hospitals escape scrutinization by not publishing statistics on their performance, especially since some statistics do not put the hospital in a favorable light. As a result of this, hospitals that are deemed to be top-notch may not be.

Number one says that *SAFETY CULTURE SCORES* reported honestly by hospital workers about what goes on in hospitals by medical/patient care teams are very important to monitor. Teams with higher scores had fewer infection problems and better patient outcomes. Than teams with lower scores.

The second idea is the use of *ONLINE DASHBOARDS* by hospitals and healthcare centers that the dashboard should list the number and types of surgical procedures with patient satisfaction surveys in a Zagat like rating system for restaurants.

Recommendation number three was the use of *OPEN NOTES*. He was referring to online doctor's notes which patients could review via the web and post comments and corrections to help the doctors and medical personnel.

Number four advocated *NO MORE GAGGING* or requiring patients to sign non-disclosure agreements about keeping silent about any medical injury. He felt that by having patients speak up, future patients would benefit.

Lastly was the idea of *USING A VIDEO CAMERA* to tape every medical procedure. He believes that this would be a great teaching tool no matter what the outcome. [xxxiii]

Some Ideas on Med Mal Caps from Senator Feinstein

In February 2004, United States Senator Dianne Feinstein had some things to say about medical malpractice.[xxxiv]

The backdrop of her remarks was a failed congressional bill favored by the Bush administration to limit non-economic damages in med mal cases covering only obstetricians and gynecologists. The cap for non-economic damages was to be $250,000.

Senator Feinstein felt that all medical specialties should be included —
not just obstetricians — with a flex cap for non-economic damages of $500,000
in a plan of her own.

One of her complaints about the bill was that it would have allowed
significant protection from medical malpractice lawsuits to drug and medical
device manufacturers — like the makers of Fen-Phen, the diet drug sensation,
and the Dalkon Shield contraceptive device. The bill would have allowed a cap
for non-economic damages against such manufacturers of $250,000, where, in
general, prior to this bill, such devices or products were not included in the
realm of medical malpractice lawsuits.

Senator Feinstein felt that, in catastrophic cases (as specified under the
language of her proposed law), the non-economic damages cap should be the
greater of $2,000,000 or $50,000 times the number of years of the life
expectancy of the victim. She said her proposal would allow for punitive
damages where proof would be below the very high standards for those to
prove fraud, oppression or malice. To qualify, a case had to pass a certain list of
questions.

What the Insurers and Physicians Groups Are Saying

Regarding changes to the MICRA cap on non-economic damages,
medical malpractice insurance carriers say that they cannot stay in the business
of providing medical malpractice insurance without premium increases if the
caps are raised. The carriers claim that they do not currently make excessive
profits underwriting medical malpractice insurance.

Physicians groups argue that doctors' fees to patients will have to go up
to cover the cost of increased premiums. They say that it will be more difficult
for them to stay in California to practice medicine if the caps are changed here.
Also, access to healthcare will diminish, especially in the State's rural areas.

These are the same arguments that prompted the passage of MICRA in
California in the first place. Note that, according to a recent study in the *New
England Journal of Medicine,* in a typical year, roughly one in fourteen physicians
faces a malpractice claim. The study also found that there is at least one med
mal claim in the career of most physicians.[xxxv]

The Rand Studies of MICRA's Effects

The Rand Corporation is a Santa Monica, California based non-profit organization that sets as its goal as "to improve policy and decision-making through research and analysis." Rand has studied MICRA for years. In their 2004 study,[xxxvi] Rand Corporation researchers analyzed 257 medical malpractice plaintiffs' verdicts in California cases from 1995 to 1999. They found:

1. That the cap on non-economic awards (commonly referred to as "pain and suffering") was imposed on 45% of the cases won by plaintiffs in the sample. Because of the cap, defendants' liabilities in those cases were reduced by an average of 30%. Death cases were capped more frequently than injury cases (58% versus 41%). According to their statistical finding, the median loss of monetary damages was minus 49% for capped cases and 28% for injury cases.

2. Plaintiffs with the most severe losses (paralysis, brain damage or a variety of other terrible losses) had their non-economic injury damage awards capped far more often than injury claims generally and had median reductions (from statistical comparisons) exceeding $1 million (compared with $286,000 for all injury cases).

3. Plaintiffs who lost the highest percentage of their total awards due to the cap were often those with injuries that led to relatively modest economic damage awards (approximately $100,000 or less) but that caused a great loss to their quality of life (as suggested by the jury's million-dollar-plus award for pain, suffering, anguish, distress, and the like). These plaintiffs sometimes received awards that were cut by two-thirds or more from the jury's original decisions.

4. Plaintiffs less than one year old had capped awards 71% of the time, compared with 41% of the time for all plaintiffs with identifiable non-fatal injuries.

In the same publication, Rand researchers stated that the cap on attorneys' fees was reduced by an average of 30% alone by the caps on fees, and 46% on average without caps on any limits. Because of the cap on attorneys' fees, the net take-home to plaintiffs was only reduced by 15%.

278

In a 2012 update on the original 2004 study,[xxxvii] the authors said that MICRA appears to have had its initial intended effect on limiting defendants' expenditures.

Additionally, Rand researchers said that, even without MICRA, medical malpractice cases have a relatively low rate of plaintiff victory at trial (22% for the plaintiffs in medical malpractice cases versus 53% in non-MICRA general injury cases) and carry high costs for expert witnesses.

Continuing, the researchers said that those with low dollar figure cases would likely find it more difficult to find representation, even with a potential high-value award from a jury for non-economic damages.

For your information, jurors cannot be told of the MICRA caps on non-economic damages. However, the attorneys, of course, do know about the caps.

According to the Rand Corporation findings, the groups that suffer the greatest losses with the current MICRA caps are the heirs of those who died from medical malpractice, and those with modest levels of economic loss. **The researchers indicated that in some cases, an allowance should be made for certain types of cases that were exceptionally tragic such as in brain damage or birth defect cases.**

Hamm, et al Study Backs Insurers & Physicians' Viewpoint

In February 2005, William G. Hamm, PhD, C. Paul Wazzan, PhD, and H. E. Frech III, PhD, co-authored a study about the economics of the MICRA reforms.[xxxviii]

The study received financial support from CAPP (Californians Allied for Patient Protection) which is actually made up of health care providers within the state.

In their report, the three economists detailed the economics of proposed California MICRA reforms. The report is favorable to healthcare providers and medical malpractice insurance carriers in California in that it supports their contentions.

Here are the objectives of the report: "Several groups and individuals have advocated for changes in MICRA, including an increase in California's $250,000 cap on non-economic damages. The purpose of this paper is to help policymakers, opinion leaders, and the public evaluate the effect of raising the MICRA cap for non-economic damages on California's healthcare system. The paper provides answers to questions left unresolved by the RAND report and other studies, such as: how does the cap affect medical malpractice insurance premiums and healthcare coverage."

The report said, "We find that the MICRA's $250,000 ceiling cap on non-economic damages has been effective in improving Californians' access to healthcare. The cap has reduced the incentive to litigate the weakest claims; it has reduced the average size of malpractice awards (i.e., severity); and it has cut total loss costs. As a result, the cap has reduced and stabilized medical malpractice insurance costs. It has discouraged unnecessary medical procedures and treatments that inflate the cost of healthcare to the consumer without improving medical outcomes.

"Our analysis concludes that an increase in the cap on awards for non-economic damages would lead to more litigation, larger awards, and higher litigation-related expenses — thereby reducing access to affordable healthcare in California. Specifically, we estimate that an increase in the cap to $500,000 would raise annual costs of California's healthcare system by an amount likely to exceed $6.5 billion.

"We also find that the cap has not markedly reduced access to the court system, especially for individuals with tenable malpractice claims."

Another finding from the report was that greater costs of healthcare resulting from a higher cap would reduce Californian's access to healthcare by making health insurance less affordable, and by reducing the number of healthcare providers, particularly in rural and low-income areas.

Their findings:

1. The MICRA cap reduces the incentive to litigate the weakest claims.

2. The potential effect of raising the cap to $500,000 or $900,000 removes the disincentive for claimants to file claims since it gives them a monetary incentive to litigate claims.

3. The MICRA cap does not restrict access to the courts.

4. The MICRA cap has reduced California's per-claim loss costs.

5. Elimination of the MICRA cap would have increased loss payments by $1.3 billion or 44% (between 1990 and 2004).

6. The MICRA cap reduces medical malpractice insurance premiums by as much as 43%.

7. California medical malpractice insurance carriers or physicians do not generate excess profits under MICRA rules.

8. An increase in the MICRA cap would cost the state healthcare system (including additional med mal insurance premiums, increased doctors' fees, and increases in healthcare insurance premiums) by $6.5 billion annually.

9. The cost of a raised cap would be borne by consumers, employers and government. A cap increase would ultimately be borne by consumers.

10. The increased healthcare costs of raising the cap would result in more Californians without any healthcare insurance, according to the authors.

11. The increased cost of healthcare with a higher cap would reduce the number of healthcare providers and might impact the number of physicians in high-risk specialties.

In short, they paint a less than rosy picture of the consequences of an increased cap.

The Hamm, et al study is supported by CAPP (Californians Allied for Patient Protection), which is actually made up of healthcare providers within the state.

In, November 2008, Hamm, et al completed a follow-up to the 2005 study just mentioned. (Hamm, William G. et al. *MICRA Lowers Healthcare Costs, Ensuring Patients Have Access to Healthcare.*) LECG, November 2008. The study was funded by CPAP.

Their primary findings were:

1. MICRA's $250,000 ceiling on non-economic damages has been effective in reducing and stabilizing medical liability insurance costs, thereby improving access to healthcare for all Californians.
2. An increase in the MICRA cap for non-economic damages would lead to more litigation, larger awards, and higher litigation related expenses.
3. We estimate that an increase in the MICRA cap for non-economic damages to $500,000 or more would raise healthcare costs in California by up to $7.9 billion annually.
4. The increase in medical liability costs resulting from a higher cap on non economic damages would be passed along to Californians attempting to use the state's healthcare system, further limiting access to the system.
5. These higher costs of healthcare would be borne by consumers who would pay more for their own healthcare costs and by federal, state and local taxpayers who would be responsible for the additional costs to cover public employees and retiree healthcare.
6. A comparison of states with and without caps on non-economic damages demonstrates that in states with caps, medical liability premiums are lower.
7. Even with the $250,000 cap on non-economic damages, the average size of all paid claims - large and small – has increased faster than the rate of inflation.
8. There is no evidence that California's cap on non-economic damages has materially reduced access to the courts for those individuals with meritorious claims of liability.
9. The MICRA cap on non-economic damages discourages unnecessary procedures and treatments that inflate the cost of healthcare to the consumer without improving patients' medical outcomes. [xxxix]

CJAC & the *Stinnett vs. Tam* Case

On January 26, 2011, Kimberly Stone, President of CJAC (the Civil Justice Association of California) through CJAC.org supported President Obama's attempts to cap non-economic damages at $250,000 for **every case of medical malpractice on a national basis**. She said that CJAC estimated that raising the cap on non-medical injuries from $250,000 to $500,000 would raise California healthcare costs by at least $9.5 billion annually (from a 2008 report by a former California non-partisan legislative analyst). According to Kimberly Stone, this increase would increase healthcare costs for a family of four in the State by $1,032 annually. [xl]

CJAC opposes those trying to weaken or eliminate MICRA. The group files actions on various other legal issues in addition to MICRA issues.

CJAC filed a brief in 2010 for Tam in *Stinnett vs. Tam*, a medical malpractice case in California, where a woman sued for loss of consortium over the death of her husband and other damages. A jury awarded her $6 million but the verdict, using the MICRA cap, was reduced to $250,000. She appealed the ruling, saying that it was no longer the 1970s when MICRA was enacted and that things are now materially different than they were in 1975.

CJAC's brief said that the courts have largely upheld MICRA and that any changes should come from the State Legislature and not the courts. [xli]

Tam prevailed in this case according to the appeals court ruling. [xlii]

Note that there have been many California MICRA-capped cases for the death of a patient. These are known as **"250 cases"** since they only pay $250,000 to the heirs of the deceased.

Other challenges to the constitutionality of MICRA have dotted the legal landscape for decades.

Case of Deceased Attorney Gary Gavello

A recent case challenging the constitutionality of MICRA that was filed in 2012 is by the family of deceased attorney Gary Gavello. Mr. Gavello died in 2008, apparently as a result of problems with post-op medications administered by anesthesiologist Bernard Millman, MD at the office of a plastic surgeon in 2008. Reportedly, a post-surgical preventable error caused the patient to stop breathing and die. Because of the MICRA cap and because the patient signed an arbitration agreement with the plastic surgeon and the nurse, the award was 20% of $250,000 or $50,000 since the plaintiff was found to be only 20% liable.

The Gavello appeal claimed that the law was unconstitutional since it denied the family the full right to a jury trial and that MICRA violates equal treatment laws since medical malpractice victims are treated differently than victims in other types of injury cases. [xliii]

Gavello's appeal was denied as the Court found that The MICRA was constitutional. [xliv]

Cases that challenge the MICRA issue that allowing only provable economic damages (such as lost wages or medical bills) severely impacts seniors who may be retired or have no income and children because they have no earnings according to Berniece Yeung.

Yeung also mentions that Bruce Brusavich, a prominent plaintiffs' malpractice attorney, feels that scarred or disfigured plaintiffs who return to the workplace are disadvantaged by the damages cap in medical malpractice cases as opposed to what such a plaintiff could recover in a non-medical malpractice case when left scarred or disfigured.

Yeung also gives space to Kathy Kneer of Planned Parenthood who believes that higher caps in The MICRA would damage a thin line of financial stability for some providers. [xlv]

Too Many Stakeholders for National Reforms?

Dan Diamond is a contributing editor to *California Healthline*, an online publication self-described as "a daily digest of news, policy and opinion." In February 2012, the californiahealthline.org site posted Diamond's article titled "Why We Can't Get National Malpractice Reform."

Diamond says that it is likely that President Obama abandoned his desire for national medical malpractice reform since the subject affects so many people who have a stake in the outcome. These include "payers, patient advocates, physicians and policymakers," Diamond writers. He points out that "All (these groups) have a different take on what national tort reform should look like."

Diamond notes that, regarding med mal improvements, one patient advocate has estimated that "a few thousand trial lawyers are blocking reform that would benefit 300 million Americans."[xlvi]

*****

As I see it, with all the fancy quantitative analysis studies mentioned above replete with charts and graphs that send a message that raised caps are bad or too expensive to bear, the authors of the reports fail to grasp and promote the reality that **medical malpractice is about a breach of trust between people, not a bunch of numbers**. What they are lacking is a thorough, comprehensive analysis which would include qualitative measures.

*****

On October 11, 2012, consumer protection activist Ralph Nader called for Governor Jerry Brown to encourage the California State Legislature to eliminate the MICRA cap for non-economic damages. Nader called the current cap "outdated and cruel," and charged that MICRA severely limits the legal rights of badly injured individuals in California and makes it extremely difficult to hold physicians and hospitals accountable for incompetent or negligent medical care. He noted that the current cap of $250,000 for pain and suffering has never been adjusted for inflation for over its thirty-five year, and that at least an increase in the cap should be made if the limit is not gotten rid of.[xlvii]

*****

Unless you have been an injured medical malpractice plaintiff, you really do not know what it is like to be screwed up by the errors of your physician — even if it only happens once in the doctor's career.

Those of you who are opposed to medical malpractice reform and favor keeping caps low for non-economic damages have no idea what you are talking about in terms of compensation for an injured person's suffering, unless you have suffered as a result of a preventable medical error.

Until then, your argument against reforming The MICRA is strictly an intellectual exercise. It's like a man trying to tell a woman who has given birth to a child what pregnancy really feels like.

*****

In death cases, brain damage cases, paralysis cases, amputation cases or cases involving other awful outcomes, an award of $250,000 for non-economic damages is an insult.

In addition, using the CPI calculator, **it would take $1,078,838.29 in today's dollars to equal $250,000 in 1975**. (The source of this figure is the CPI Inflation Calculator. *CPI* means *consumer price index.*).

Here's another problem with The MICRA. If periodic payments are made under a settlement of a MICRA case, there is no provision for the cost of increased future care via inflation — unless it is specified in any settlement.

*****

When the injuries of human beings are part of the picture, we need to consider more than just numbers.

Looking over the research I had gathered, the heavy hitters in the California medical malpractice insurance business seemed to be coming on too strong for my tastes. I got the feeling that something important was being buried but I couldn't put my finger on it...

I was tired of looking at numbers, projections, hypotheses and graphs and the like. I was just about to conclude my search for information regarding medical malpractice reform. Then I made one last pass on the subject on Amazon.com and found a book titled *The Medical Malpractice Myth* **by Tom Baker.**[xlviii]

*****

Tom Baker, an attorney and a law professor, whose father and father-in-law are both MDs, was uniquely qualified to write his book.

In December 2005 when the book was first published, Mr. Baker was the Director of the Insurance Law Center at the University of Connecticut. He is currently a Professor of Law and Health Sciences at the University of Pennsylvania Law School. Baker is also a consultant to insurance companies and law firms. He is an expert about insurance law and has some provocative thoughts about medical malpractice reforms.

An Epidemic of What?

In the course of writing his book, Mr. Baker poured over hundreds of printed sources: annual reports, industry reports, financial disclosures books, articles, and memos and the like. It is fair to say that he gave documentation and evidence to back up everything he wrote. He lists hundreds of citations in his bibliography. All of it befits the expert that he is.

In *The Medical Malpractice Myth*, **Mr. Baker gives clear and convincing evidence that there is an epidemic of medical malpractice in this country but not an epidemic of medical malpractice lawsuits — in spite of what some politicians and med mal insurance carriers and physician groups would have you believe.**

He does not buy the argument that there is a medical malpractrice insurance crisis. He offers up that most of the time, the crises of the past were due to the unique cyclical nature of the medical malpractice insurance business.

The **arguments against** medical malpractice reform in California seemed **less credible** to me from Baker's findings.

Baker studied numerous published reports about medical malpractice to arrive at his findings. He found that, over the course of time, the number of medical malpractice claims has remained as a stable percentage of all medical care. Hence, there is no "epidemic" of medical malpractice claims.

Mr. Baker estimates that for every case of medical malpractice that is reported (using reviews of hospital records) somewhere between *four and seven times* more malpractice cases go unreported. The reviews he used were conducted independently by different researchers in different decades: the 1970s, 1980s, 1990s and the early 21st century. He names the studies and the evidence he presents is convincing.

From his book he noted that, "In the mid-1970s, the California Hospital and Medical Association sponsored a study on medical malpractice that they expected would support their tort reform efforts. But to their surprise and dismay, the study showed that medical malpractice injured tens of thousands of people every year — more than automobile and workplace accidents. The study also showed that, despite the rhetoric, most of the victims did not sue. But almost nobody heard about the study because the associations decided that these facts conflicted with their tort reform message."

The cover-up has continued to the present day.

Medical malpractice insurance carriers and their supporters don't want the general public to know that *there is an epidemic of medical malpractice but not an epidemic of medical malpractice lawsuits.*

How Med Mal Insurers Are Different

Baker points out why medical malpractice insurance companies are different from other types of insurance companies, especially liability insurance companies (auto and homeowner insurance companies).

Liability insurers know that once a year passes from the date of a potential liability situation when a claim is made on a policy in force, if a claim is not made, the injured party cannot sue due to a statute of limitations. (One exception to that might be because of fraud.) Also, the great majority of liability claims are settled without unreasonable delays — thus closing the books quickly.

This is *not* the case with medical malpractice claims.

Baker says that with medical malpractice claims, it can be several years from the date of malpractice before a claim is made. Why? **Because the malpractice may not be discovered right away.**

Also, due to the fact that some claims can be paid over time if they exceed a certain dollar figure, an older policy can have losses against it for several years. So, the premiums collected from several years prior, in total, may not amount to enough "reserves" against losses. If financial reserves get too low, state regulators can take over an insurance carrier if the reserves are not increased to acceptable levels.

Ideally, reserves should be set based upon a realistic estimate of a potential payout. According to insurance company accounting rules, these reserves are treated as losses or expenses against income from the premiums.

This might leave a medical malpractice insurer short of money to cover its losses since they have tried to remain competitive with lower pricing to keep market share. Then, in fact, they got hammered by claims from prior years. Pricing in the med mal insurance business is made by "best guess" estimates and is an art not a science. At least that was the case when Baker wrote his book.

Further exacerbating the situation, if the investments an insurance company makes turn sour, the insurer may have to raise prices to cover those losses which affect whether or not the insurer has enough capital reserves. If the stock market or bond market turn down for an extended period of time, here come the premium increases.

These situations usually result in significant increases. These "jolts" to the cost of medical malpractice insurance can result in a so-called malpractice insurance "crises" for doctors. It should be noted that these "jolts" usually impact the physicians in the higher risk areas of medicine, like neurosurgery and obstetrics, more than other specialties, according to Baker.

In other words, the nature of medical malpractice insurance companies is that they are more "cyclical" than liability insurers. Thus, doctors sometimes cry foul and claim a "medical malpractice insurance crisis" when in fact there is none. It is just the nature of the business and the need for a price increase.

According to the evidence Baker presents, these "crises" occurred in the 1970s, 1980s, and 1990s and early in the 21st century. He also says, that the cycles will continue in the future all else being equal.

Creating a System to Share Errors

Baker believes that autonomy, or the freedom from restrictive regulation, is part of our "value set" in this country. Taking away the right to sue impinges on that value set. People in America want the right to sue if they have been injured. Whether or not they sue, they want that right.

On the other hand, softening the financial blow for a doctor or other healthcare provider who owns up to their mistakes is also deemed acceptable to people who are asked to judge such cases.

Interestingly, Baker pointed out that, as a group, anesthesiologists once paid high premiums for medical malpractice insurance relative to all medical specialties. In an effort to improve the overall care offered by anesthesiologists and thus reduce the incidence of malpractice among their specialty, they shared information about their mistakes with each other, and developed new products and procedures to make it safer for patients to undergo general anesthesia. It worked. The incidence of medical malpractice against anesthesiologists dropped and their medical malpractice premiums are now in a mid-range compared to all medical specialties instead of being at the high end.

Baker advocates using a reporting agency for all incidents of medical malpractice so that all doctors can learn from errors. His choice would be a state agency, like the department of public health, since physicians as a whole have shown a disinclination to monitor or police themselves on their own. He makes a sound argument for the benefits of such a system. He suggests monetary penalties for non-compliance, severe penalties.

Keep Medical Devices Out of the Med Mal Arena

Surprisingly, **Baker offers evidence that medical device manufacturers are quite fond of the idea of having claims against them classified as medical malpractice claims.**

With caps for non-economic damages set low by law, manufacturers of faulty medical devices could dodge the bullet of large tort claims if medical product failures ever fall under medical malpractice laws.

This is clearly a backdoor attempt to hoodwink the general public since **medical malpractice has to do with *standard of care* and not medical devices**. A bad medical device is a bad medical device is a bad medical device, not bad care.

The medical device lobby would love to have our Congress enact laws to include medical devices under the umbrella of medical malpractice.

In my opinion, it is a terrible idea and one that may be used to confuse the issue of an epidemic of medical malpractice claims. This is one reason why we shouldn't have Congress get involved in medical malpractice reform. Cases like the Dalkon Shield debacle and Fen-Phen should not be in the medical malpractice arena, in my opinion. That would promote bad or substandard medical devices. You might have to think about that for a moment.

If you haven't figured it out, if a bad device like that makes it on the market and lawsuits are filed because it injures patients, and such cases fall under the prevailing medical malpractice laws (with low caps for non-economic damages), a manufacturer of such a device won't be penalized nearly enough in a monetary sense, in my opinion, as it might be under normal tort recovery laws.

It should be noted that medical malpractice torts rank third nationally, behind automobile liability torts and workers comp tort claims. If the real aim of lawmakers is tort reform, it shouldn't begin with med mal insurance reforms but with tort reforms for auto liability and workers comp reforms.

More "Defensive Medicine"?

Medical societies and med mal insurance companies also like to raise the issue that physicians will practice *defensive medicine* in the face of the specter of medical malpractice. This is so untrue.

As Baker points out, research shows that while there may be defensive medicine to some degree, the impact on overall healthcare costs is very small. Doctors order certain tests, order consultations with specialists, and perform certain procedures in the great majority of cases only if there are clinical indications for doing so, not to cover their behinds. Yet physicians and the general public see defensive medicine as being very costly when it is not. It makes up a very small fraction of overall healthcare costs.

Possible Shortage of Physicians?

Another part of the med mal myth is that raising medical malpractice insurance premiums will reduce the number of doctors to care for patients. It is simply not true.

Baker says that there's something else that is really happening in some parts of the country. That is, in areas with significant population increases, there are fewer doctors per person. Doctors coming in to practice medicine in those geographic areas lag behind population growth.

Where healthcare insurance coverage is not as easily available, doctors do not want to practice in those areas. So, shortages can occur. Those tend to be rural areas. Also, most doctors will tell you that they prefer urban areas to rural areas, so fewer doctors go to rural areas.

Over time, the number of doctors in this country has increased, even though med mal insurance premiums have gone up. At one time, the projected glut of doctors was substantial so the amount of federal funding for training physicians fell. What eventually happened was that due to reduced funding for physician training, shortages of physicians in some parts of the United States occurred. These shortages were not the result of rising medical malpractice insurance premiums due to med mal lawsuits.

Openness Could Reduce Injuries and Lawsuits

According to Baker's research, medical malpractice mistakes by doctors and healthcare professionals kill more people in the United States than auto liability accidents and workers comp accidents do combined.

Professor Baker states his case for sharing information in the medical care arena as a means to reduce preventable medical mistakes that kill and injure people. He espoused this before Marty Makary wrote his book in 2012.

Tom Baker believes that reporting of all medical malpractice incidents is good for patients and medical professionals and their malpractice insurers.

When a patient is injured via malpractice by a doctor, hospital or other medical care provider, there is **a moral imbalance** between the two sides. A lawsuit is the means we have in this country to correct the imbalance. It also allows the patient to find out what went wrong.

Research uncovered by Baker showed that doctors who explained the risks of medical procedures or treatments, and were honest when things went wrong demonstrated to their patients that they cared. This boded well for doctors at trial as juries tended to be more forgiving to doctors who accepted moral responsibility. Many injured patients, under these conditions, chose not to sue once they were informed. On the opposite side of the coin, when the patient did not find out what happened, they sued not only for damages but to find out what had happened.

A Solution for Smaller Claims

Baker is against low and unrealistic caps for non-economic damages to patients injured by malpractice.

Professor Baker offers evidence that those most seriously injured and those with low value claims are hurt the most by potentially low non-economic damage caps. By shutting off the avenue of tort recovery to these patients, it handcuffs their freedom and takes away their justice. It makes them bear the heaviest burdens when malpractice occurs.

For lower value or smaller claims, Baker offers a system along the lines of "no-fault" insurance. All that is needed is an objective finding of

294

malpractice (violation of a standard of care) according to medical records and a resulting injury. At that point, with an admission by the at-fault party/parties and an apology, a settlement could be negotiated with an insurer based upon certain guidelines — thus saving both sides costly litigation expenses and offering incentives to both to settle the smaller claims quickly. For me, it was thought-provoking to read it.

Since a certain standard of proof is needed, this by itself would keep phony claims from clogging the system. There must be a breach of the standard of care and causation or a claim does not qualify. So much for "nuisance" claims getting paid.

Also, Baker makes it very clear that he does not advocate "no fault" medical malpractice insurance for all claims. He believes that the larger claims involving the most serious injuries need to be adjudicated by the courts.

Enter the PPHRA

Baker lays it all out in his **Patient Protection Healthcare Responsibility Act (PPHRA)**. It gives a detailed explanation of what is needed for real comprehensive reforms. I'll try to highlight and summarize what he said.

Tom Baker hammers home **four key findings** in his book.

First, since research shows that there is too much medical malpractice, **the first goal of any effective medical malpractice reform should be to reduce the incidence of medical malpractice.**

Second, many injured patients cannot tell if medical malpractice occurred to themselves. Because of that, **patients need information so that they can determine if medical malpractice occurred.**

Third, most people injured by medical malpractice are not compensated. Therefore, any real **malpractice reform should have a mechanism for all injured patients to obtain compensation for their injuries** — if that is their wish.

Fourth, the boom and bust insurance cycle of the medical malpractice carriers causes the medical malpractice insurance crises that are particularly hard on doctors over time. Therefore, **moderating the effect of the insurance cycle should be a goal of malpractice reform**.

Chapter 19 lays out Baker's plan in detail.

*****

Hopefully, this chapter and the preceding chapter are representative of the overall thinking about the current medical malpractice laws. This is a heavily debated topic, so it was only possible to include a small sampling of the discourse on medical malpractice reform.

Chapter 19—Mechanism for No-Fault Malpractice Reform

In order to give you more details about the **Patient Protection and Healthcare Responsibility Act (PPHRA)** proposed by Professor Tom Baker, I've included significant ideas in this chapter that Baker has offered up. For a full course on what he has to say, refer to his book, *The Medical Malpractice Myth*.[xlix]

The PPHRA has four parts. It is proposed as legislation for any state that wants to adopt it.

Part One espouses an open and honest medical-injury disclosure and enforcement process to reduce the number of patient injuries over time.

Part Two suggests an offer of apology and restitution for the wrongdoing and a procedure for settling some medical malpractice lawsuits.

Part Three discusses a no-fault patient compensation insurance program, with moderate benefits, as a supplement to current medical malpractice insurance.

The fourth part strongly suggests a different type of insurance to protect doctors and other licensed healthcare providers who need malpractice insurance from the worst effects of the medical malpractice insurance cycle.

Baker believes that his proposed recommendations will lead to more realistic reforms than the current med mal tort reform proposals (which mostly focus on cap limits, a very shallow view of medical malpractice reform).

*****

PART ONE

Baker's plan requires that **every healthcare practitioner** working on a patient inform the patient (or whoever is responsible for the patient), both orally and in writing, whenever it can be determined that a patient has suffered an adverse healthcare event.

A severe penalty would be imposed for non-disclosure up to and including loss of license.

The proposed Act requires **reporting the adverse event or possible adverse healthcare event to the Department of Public Health (DPH) and the health insurance company or entity paying for the affected patient's healthcare**.

The DPH would make information from the reports available to the public to promote patient-safety research and awareness by use of a required audit on patient files.

Rather than guessing about causation, Baker believes that it is better to inform if the possibility exists rather than waiting. He believes that the same holds true if the medical management of a case may have caused a problem or made an injury worse.

How can anyone argue with the propostion that patients are entitled to know what happened to them when the result is not what their doctors intended?

According to Baker, The American Medical Association medical ethics code requires doctors to tell their patients about both good and bad outcomes. A doctor is ethically required by the AMA to inform a patient about everything necessary for the patient to understand what went wrong when something does go wrong. However, it is not the law.

According to Baker's research, the evidence showed that, by the late 1990s, doctors were not fully disclosing injuries no matter if they were preventable or not.

Thus, Baker developed his PPHRA. Baker included all healthcare professionals as being obligated to report **in writing** adverse outcomes to a patient, not just doctors. His proposal means that a senior professional will be less likely to silence lower-ranking professionals involved in the care.

PPHRA's reporting requirement is included so adverse events can be used to improve public safety.

With an admission of negligence, and a severe penalty for ignoring that, it is hoped that those under the spotlight will not withhold information about bad outcomes. Of course, the proposed law will not stop human nature in not wanting to report a bad outcome.

Baker states that **expecting healthcare professionals to disclose adverse events by self-regulation has been a failure**.

PART TWO

Baker promotes the idea that the Act would create a **new apology and restitution procedure** that would give medical malpractice insurance companies, healthcare providers defending themselves and patients an incentive to settle cases before going to trial.

*****

According to a *Wall Street Journal* article by writer Laura Landro,[1] she pointed out that when a medical malpractice injury occurs, doctors want to apologize. However, they are led to believe that it could end up as a financial disaster when just the opposite is true.

The article goes on to say that at the University of Michigan Health System, new policies that fully disclosed malpractice injuries to patients were implemented. In addition, apologies were given when merited. After implementation, the **number of pre-suit claims and the number of lawsuits themselves — combined — dropped dramatically between 2001 and 2007**.

*****

Returning to Baker, he says that medical care professionals who apologize and acknowledge fault would be able to offer restitution for an injury

299

within a reasonable time — after it becomes possible to know the extent of the patient's injuries and future losses. The apology would be an admission of liability.

A patient would then have a reasonable time to consider whether to accept the offer. A rejection of any offer sends the case to trial with the only question being the amount of the patient's damages.

A 1994 New Jersey initiative for cases involving clear liability contained the idea of an "offer of judgment." A reduction in the size of any settlement is the hoped for outcome in clear liability claim payments for insurers by using the apology and restitution portion of Baker's plan. The restitution portion of this is the "offer of judgment."

Baker shows that, in a large number of closed claims where liability was clear, insurance payouts were higher than in cases where liability was not so clear. Baker also noted that insurance company executives recognized that some cases had clear liability. So, he offered up his thinking for those types of cases.

Medical malpractice insurance claims in clear liability cases drain the coffers of medical malpractice insurers more than other types of med mal claims. Wouldn't that lead forward-thinking managers at such insurance companies to seek a way to reduce those kinds of payments?

That is what Baker hopes the **apology and restitution provison of his proposed law** will do. He offers the results of research he did to support his position. This is similar to an "offer of judgment rule" common in federal court and some state courts. The apology idea comes from Baker.

Normally, where the "offer of judgment rule" applies in federal cases, consequences are usually negligible. Court costs do not ordinarily include attorney fees, and therefore the offer-of-judgment rule does not give a defendant the possibility of recovering attorneys' fees from a plaintiff who turns down a good offer.

Baker thinks that one should not have a hard time believing that applying Taft's proposal would have a much larger effect on medical malpractice claims since they are larger and require more legal time on both sides to settle. As a result, there might be more room to reduce payouts if both sides have an incentive such as the ones just mentioned.

*****

Under Baker's PPHRA proposal, plaintiffs who reject an offer of restitution have to pay the defendant's attorney fees — **unless** the jury award is at least 20% *more* than the defendant's offer. Baker's approach makes it much more likely that plaintiffs will have to pay the defendant's fees, and therefore increases the incentive to accept the restitution offer.

When a medical error is undisclosed to and later discovered by a plaintiff, it can break the trust between a doctor and a patient. It is the lack of apology that really disrupts this trust, according to Baker and can lead to lawsuits.

With the proposed apology and restitution, a repair in the break becomes possible. This makes it highly possible that the offer will be accepted in a medical malpractice case, more than in the auto and homeowners' cases Professor Baker studied.

According to Baker, based upon Taft's own experience with medical malpractice lawsuits and on research on the effect of apologies in malpractice lawsuits, Taft argues that doctors should be willing to apologize even without an incentive.

Baker notes that Lee Taft found in his own jury research that juries awarded lower damages in cases in which the doctor apologized and showed genuine remorse. Further, other research showed that plaintiffs were also willing to accept smaller settlements in the situation where an apology was offered.

Because fear and distrust have built up among doctors and their defense lawyers over time, an incentive to apologize probably is necessary in Baker's opinion.

Briefly, many plaintiff's attorneys do not like Baker's idea about making an apology saying it is too one-sided.

What Baker wants to promote is that **research shows that plaintiffs want more than money. They want to know what happened and seek closure and a sincere apology.**

*****

Baker's main objective here is to illustrate the difference between evidence-based medical liability reform and the tort reform ideas that emerge from medical malpractice myths.

His core concept in medical malpractice tort reform is to base reform on evidence over time. He says that doing so will lead to achieving goals on lawsuit deterrence, compensation, and corrective justice goals.

*****

PART THREE

Baker offers a **no-fault program** with modest benefits principally intended to provide compensation for, and incentives to avoid, injuries that are "moderate."

Any patient injured by an adverse healthcare event would be entitled to compensation for that injury for activities that an injured patient cannot perform due to the injury from insurance purchased by the responsible healthcare provider(s), according to a schedule established by the Department of Public Health. The schedule would compensate patients for: reasonable healthcare and rehabilitation expenses not covered by other insurance or benefit plans, lost wages or patient services for activities which the patient can no longer perform that are not recoverable from other sources, and up to a maximum amount for an adverse event (or series of related events).

The size of the maximum amount would be set by the legislature, say from $50,000 to $80,000 in Baker's mind.

Additionally, a minimal interference with the current tort approach would be ideal, saving the plaintiff and defendant insurance carriers money for those cases where there is clear liability.

The DPH would establish a procedure for eligibility and compensation, modeled on workers' compensation and Social Security benefit procedures. Patients would be allowed to have the assistance of an attorney or patient advocate at any hearing, at their own expense. State-paid advocates would be available for patients with earnings below a certain amount.

Baker observes that no-fault compensation for medical negligence injuries turns out to be an idea that many like in theory, but almost no one likes in practice.

Healthcare providers favor no-fault in theory since it feels less adversarial and more consistent with the therapeutic nature of their calling. But, in the real world, it threatens to open a floodgate of claims and dramatically increase their insurance premiums.

Baker offers that **workers comp accidents injure far fewer people than medical malpractice. Yet, workers' compensation insurance premiums in the United States for 2003 were five times as large as medical malpractice insurance premiums.**

Patient advocates like no-fault in theory since it offers a promise of quick, no-hassle compensation. In practice, once they realize that they have to prove that medical treatment caused the patients' injuries, it is unfavorable. Added to that is the idea that no-fault damages are not enough to pay for the skilled advocates and experts needed to overcome healthcare providers' causation defenses in serious-injury cases.

Tom Baker asserts that medical negligence injuries are quite different from workplace accidents, so workers' compensation may be a poor model. Workers know what to expect in the workplace and have a good idea of what happened to them in a workplace accident. If they do not know, they usually have ways to find out. Patients do not.

Two very limited no-fault medical-injury programs exist in the United States, one in Virginia and one in Florida. Both apply only to a narrow range of birth injuries. Neither is widely regarded as a success.

*****

Why include a no-fault compensation concept in PPHRA?

First, no-fault contrasts the American Medical Association position that tort liability should be cut back since tort lawsuits do not offer enough to injured patients. Yet, they offer no proposal to increase the number of patients who should be compensated.

In comparison to the Virginia and Florida birth injury programs, Baker's no-fault compensation would be most important for medical injuries that are ignored by medical malpractice lawyers today.

Birth injury cases draw lots of attention from hungry lawyers. Lower value claims do not.

A no-fault system, in Baker's eyes, might help obstetricians and other high-risk medical professionals attain better risk management outcomes akin to what anesthesiologists, as a group, attained over time.

Baker's no-fault proposal puts forth streamlined administrative rules to compensate lower value claims. Closed claim research Baker uncovered shows that **claims worth less than $200,000 are seldom pursued by plaintiff attorneys**.

Baker offers that medical negligence injuries, auto liability injuries, and workers comp injuries depict how severe they are in a pyramid-like formation — with many lower-value injuries at the bottom and fewer serious injuries at the top. **Professor Baker says that med mal lawsuits ignore about 75% of the actual number of med mal injuries which could be claimed. He wants more focus on the 75%.**

Would this require a massive tort replacement program?

No. A small supplemental program is envisioned with a maximum award in the $50,000 to $80,000 range. However, in my mind, it needs to be up to $200,000 for a maximum award and should start at about $30,000.

This could enable an injured patient with a $250,000 claim to settle for $200,000 without the colossal hassle of a full-blown lawsuit, which is expensive and distasteful.

Giving up tort liability for high-value medical malpractice claims would be a very bad idea, both in Baker's and my way of thinking.

The thinking centers around the difficulty and expense of proving causation, as opposed to doing so in a workplace injury case. Remember, patients do not have open access to the medical evidence of a healthcare provider's negligence. Filing suit may be the only way to get to the truth, which is sometimes covered up even when records are available.

In workplace injury cases, discovering the truth may be a lot easier by comparison.

Until there is a solid track record for medical malpractice no-fault, a comprehensive tort replacement program will be dead-on-arrival in any legislature in any state of the country in Baker's mind.

*****

PART FOUR

Professor Baker thinks hospitals, nursing homes, rehabilitation centers, surgery centers and similar facilities should obtain liability insurance (or comparable protection) for all licensed healthcare providers who provide care services using the organization's facilities. This "**enterprise insurance**" would cover traditional tort claims and it would also provide the patient-compensation benefits described previously in PART THREE.

Doctors with office and hospital practices would need their own medical liability insurance policies to cover their office practice, under Baker's plan.

Serious medical malpractice suits (including OB or neurosurgery cases) usually involve services that are provided in a hospital or similar facility. This means that, with enterprise insurance, premiums for personal medical liability insurance of a doctor with a substantial hospital practice would be much less than it is now, even with the new patient-compensation benefits.

Enterprise Insurance

Tom Baker's *enterprise insurance* concept in the PPHRA is his answer to the medical malpractice insurance crisis. It obligates hospitals and similar organizations to provide insurance covering all liabilities arising out of services performed, or to be performed, in their facilities.

True *enterprise liability* (the organization being ultimately liable for medical mistakes) has not caught on. Truth be known, hospitals and HMOs resisted taking over liability from doctors and doctors resisted giving it up. Doctors were afraid that giving up liability would mean losing control over patient care.

Enterprise insurance offers many of the benefits of enterprise liability, but without asking doctors to give up liability or patient care control. Baker says that, in this scenario, all the hospital or other enterprise has to do is provide insurance.

Liability continues to rest firmly on the doctors' shoulders (except, of course, for mistakes by hospital personnel). Since the hospital has to pay for the doctors' insurance, it has a bigger incentive to design systems so that doctors make fewer mistakes, and so the mistakes that do happen have less serious results.

Enterprise insurance also makes more sense than individualized insurance as a strategy for dealing with the ugly reality of insurance underwriting cycle problems discussed in Baker's book. The individualized approach places too much of the burden of rapid premium increases on doctors in high-risk specialties and in high-risk locations. Enterprise insurance shifts the burden of rapid and unpredictable insurance price increases to organizations better equipped to manage them.

In Baker's mind, hospitals, nursing homes, rehab centers, and other large healthcare facilities provide a more diversified range of services than doctors and, thus, face more diversified risks. This greater diversity allows hospitals to spread the cost of liability insurance across both high-risk and low-risk services, so that the burden of suddenly increased premiums would not fall on a narrow range of higher-risk services, like obstetrical care.

In the real world, some medical schools and some HMOs and hospitals already provide liability insurance for their doctors. As these organizations have learned, they are better able to manage the volatility of insurance premiums than doctors making alternative arrangements in difficult market conditions.

What are the *objections* to enterprise insurance?

One objection is that enterprise insurance would interfere with the healthcare market, and this may well be the easiest concern to answer. Given the superior ability of hospitals and other health organizations to obtain medical liability insurance, it is surprising that these organizations have not already assumed that responsibility on behalf of all doctors who use their facilities.

Did you know that federal anti-kickback law prevents hospitals from paying doctors to bring patients to the hospital?

The idea is that doctors should pick hospitals based on their best medical judgement, not on the share of the hospital bill or other benefits that the hospital is willing to kick back to the doctor.

This may be one reason why enterprise insurance has not caught on. Because of this law, there is real concern that **voluntarily** providing liability insurance to doctors would be an illegal kickback, unless the doctors are hospital employees.

*****

Proximate to the publication of Baker's book in 2005, during one medical malpractice insurance crisis, there were some hospitals wanting to provide insurance to private doctors in order to make sure that the physicians could afford to keep practicing in the hospital. Those hospitals filed special requests with the U.S. Department of Health and Human Services to make sure that providing the insurance would not get them in trouble under the anti-kickback law. HHS gave the hospitals "advisory opinions" allowing them to provide the insurance but pretty much nixed the idea of allowing it all the time.

*****

Professor Baker feels that a state law requiring hospitals to provide liability insurance to doctors would completely eliminate the risk of federal prosecution for giving insurance to doctors. If every hospital within a state *had* to provide the insurance, then the insurance would not affect the doctors' choices about which hospital to use. On the other hand, it might make hospitals choosier about which doctors they allow to use their facilities. That would be a very good thing. It would force many doctors to improve their skill levels and the quality of their patient care efforts.

If legal liability remains with the doctor, and not the organization, it helps the doctor retain moral authority over patient care. Baker says that there will be conflicts between doctors and the institutions that provide their insurance, but enterprise insurance gives doctors more autonomy than would enterprise liability.

Baker also believes that the large numbers of doctors who already get their insurance through hosptials, HMOs, and medical schools are not rushing out to buy their own insurance. He feels that they seem to be managing fine with this privately arranged form of enterprise insurance.

Objections about administrative complications of a new system almost always are "makeweight arguments." They are promoted to hide the less popular interest-based objections, and this enterprise insurance situation is no exception. Insurance companies that sell insurance mainly to doctors surely will oppose enterprise insurance, as will some hospitals.

What the big insurance carriers want to avoid is losing doctors' insurance business, while hospitals want to avoid the additional expenses of more insurance. Those will be the real motives involved in blocking such ideas.

Before such ideas can be put into the real world, many important details need to be worked out such as who pays for what kinds of claims, who is covered by what liability policy and the like. Perhaps heated disagreements will be the norm early on, but then the parties involved will find solutions if it is the law.

*****

As one can see, this PPHRA plan suggests a completely different approach to medical liability reform than the damage caps do. This approach would compensate more patients who are injured by medical injuries and keep out "invalid" claims.

The thinking is that medical liabiility insurance may cost more after a proposal like Baker's is passed into law. However, we would have safer healthcare, better compensation for patient injuries, and a fairer distribution of insurance premiums.

Such a law would only cost more from the perspective of medical providers. Baker's proposal would shift more injury costs to organizations that are in a good position to prevent injuries in the first place. That should cut costs, not increase them, he says.

Would you prefer evidence-based medical malpractice insurance reform or myth-based reform?

Baker's PPHRA is evidence-based, as you have seen. It is based upon real information, not perpetual myths. If you want more detail, read his book *The Medical Malpractice Myth*.

In contrast, the tort reform proposals that emerge out of the medical malpractice myth stand in sharp contrast.

In 2005, the White House proposed curbing lawsuit abuse with needed medical liability reform. The reform included: (1) imposing a $250,000 cap on non-economic damages, (2) unspecified limits on punitive damages, (3) eliminating lump-sum damage awards in favor of periodic payments, (4) shortening the period after an injury in which a patient might bring a claim, and (5) eliminating the legal rule that makes each defendant responsible for all of the harm in the event that the other defendants do not have enough insurance or money to pay for their share.

With one exception, the White House proposals had at that time a clear and well-targeted aim: to reduce the number of high-severity, high-damage malpractice lawsuits, and to reduce the amount of damages that a severely injured patient could collect.

The one exception was the punitive-damages proposal. In the real world, punitive-damage reform does not have very much to do with true medical malpractice lawsuits, which almost never involve punitive damages.

It seems clear to me that what the Bush administration wanted to hide was that drug companies and medical device manufacturers were the real constituency for Bush's punitive-damages reform, *not* doctors and hospitals.

A federal law would have been introduced to make medical malpractice claims include ethical prescription drugs and medical devices like the Dalcon Shield, which are not currently a part of medical malpractice laws.

This would have been a quick and dirty way to appease many wealthy companies that offer products which have injured thousands causing many individuals to sue them. Or rather, their liability insurance carriers.

What Dalcon and the drug makers who were sued should have done was to offer good products and not harmful ones.

310

Baker talks about the American tort system being carefully honed from years of court cases and that Americans do not want to give up the right to sue. It has become a part of our culture.

Tom Baker does not advocate giving up that right, and neither do I. In cases like the Dalcon Shield case and cases involving harmful ethical drugs, we need to have the right to sue — period. Otherwise, companies that offer such defective products will not be held accountable and escape high-dollar tort claims when they should be warranted.

None of the Bush White House proposals would have improved the accuracy of malpractice claiming, increased the number of injured patients who would be compensated, or improved patient safety. Not one of the Bush White House proposals would have protected doctors from the next medical malpractice insurance crisis or provided real, immediate relief for doctors who deliver babies. What they would have done, instead, was increase patients' share of the medical malpractice burden.

Baker believes non-reporting does nothing to improve patient safety. He feels that too many patients are not paid for medical negligence injuries, and this belief is based on research spanning over four decades at least. He has shown that patients hear about what happened to them far too late in the process to their detriment. Lastly, he offers that doctors are asked to bear too much of the medical liability insurance burden.

To address the real problems, he believes that the medical malpractice laws should start with the evidence, not myths.

Chapter 20—What I'd Like to See Happen

After considerable thought, here is what I would like to see happen to MICRA and the reporting of medical malpractice cases.

Members of several patient rights groups who did not wish to be named generally agreed with what I have to say in this chapter and offered no additional thoughts.

I want to see a system for settling lower value med mal claims put into law and practice. Many attorneys in this state will not take a case with a value under $200,000. Therefore, a "no-fault" or lower value claims adjudication system for claims up to $200,000 is needed, and it would provide potential liberty and justice for all. Set the bar at a minimum of say $30,000 and an upper limit of $200,000. This would be advantageous to injured plaintiffs in that they would not have to shell out big money to hire an attorney since it would be based upon a **clear negligence finding either by mutual agreement or a judicial ruling**. In such cases, the only decision is how much is the value of the claim. These cases should fall under special rules in the Superior Court of California with a ceiling on each case of $200,000. This system could be added on to The MICRA after some thoughtful development. Still, I think that this may be difficult to achieve since it is theoretical and will significantly increase the number of claims. But, it is the wave of the future. Tom Baker laid out a framework for this. This would provide justice for the 80+% of preventable medical malpractice injuries that are currently uncompensated in this state.

The MICRA caps of $250,000 for non-economic damages need to be higher. I advocate raising the MICRA cap for non-economic damages implemented in 1975 to $1,000,000. The rate of inflation has increased by over 320% since 1975. That means that you need more than $1,000,000 today to be equal to the purchasing power of $250,000 in 1975 when The MICRA became law.

For someone like me who had one of the most painful and invasive surgeries on earth due to gross negligence malpractice, $250,000 is chump change. In my case or others where one or more additional surgeries might be required in the future, a higher cap on non-economic damages could be used for future pain and suffering in addition to the pain already suffered. In such cases, $250,000 is insufficient.

It may be time to legislate Tom Baker's idea of *Enterprise Insurance* to provide adequate levels of insurance along with the increased caps.

My contention is that MICRA rewards bad medical care. By capping non-economic damages, medical malpractice insurance companies pay out less money and then they charge physicians less than they otherwise would for med mal insurance premiums. Doctors are the beneficiaries of lower medical malpractice insurance premiums. Because the settlements are lower, agencies like the Medical Board of California do not look at errant physicians as critically as they might otherwise. Doctors benefit in this way by escaping more severe penalties that the Medical Board of California can order.

Lower payouts result when out-of-court settlements are encouraged for injured plaintiffs who do not have the finances to go to trial. This favors doctors and the reduced medical malpractice premiums they will pay. Lower payouts mean medical malpractice insurance premiums will be less likely to rise or will not go up significantly, unless insurers in California are caught in the insurance cycle.

Doctors benefit when smaller cases are discouraged. Without a case, there's no payout, and when many smaller cases don't move forward, there's no rise in medical malpractice insurance premiums. Also, it is not likely that a case that goes unfiled will receive much scrutiny from the Medical Board of California regarding actions against the errant doctor.

I favor a gradual increase to raise the MICRA caps. This would counteract the "knee-jerk" of rapidly rising medical malpractice premiums. I suggest raising the cap up by **$75,000 per year** until a new $1,000,000 cap is reached, in this case ten years. After that, on every fifth anniversary of reaching the $1,000,000 cap, the law should be reviewed and possibly adjusted upward but *never* lowered. That would allow med mal insurance carriers to fill their coffers against future liability that is sure to come before the higher caps become law.

In cases where the plaintiff has an awful outcome like paralysis or brain damage, I favor a non-economic damages cap of up to $4 million. Severely injured patients should be eligible to collect much higher amounts for

313

non-economic injuries. A "one size fits all" limit does not seem realistic at all. Families of severely injured plaintiffs suffer tremendously trying to care for severely injured family members. They need all the money that they can get to care for their injured loved ones.

If a patient dies from medical malpractice, the death benefit should be at least $500,000. No ifs, ands or buts here. Wrongful death verdicts for plaintiffs can bring millions in civil cases. One million dollars would be even better.

I favor implementing the suggestions put forth by Dr. Marty Makary as far as improving patient safety. Why? His ideas are based on years of experience as a surgeon. Embracing them will likely result in fewer medical malpractice injuries because they make sense. I do not propose that these ideas need to be in a series of laws. Rather, they need to be adopted in the day to day practice of medicine.

I favor Tom Baker's evidence-based reform idea of reporting all medical malpractice injuries to a state organization like the Department of Public Health. The potential benefits seem obvious and were discussed at length in the last chapter. We need evidence-based reform to destroy common misconceptions about medical malpractice. This is how it should start.

The Medical Board of California needs to be more on the side of consumer advocacy and less on the side of a physician majority. If that is not possible, the Board needs to be abolished and a new medical watchdog agency needs to be established.

From what I learned in my research, the Medical Board of California seems guided in too many ways by a physician majority. It protects bad physicians all too easily. As a result, patient care suffers. This needs to be changed. The Board needs to police its physicians.

The Medical Board of California has not lived up to its original purpose. It seems that this may be changing for the better based on the recent letter from Senator Price, Jr. and Assemblyman Gordon to the Director of the Medical Board of California which was discussed earlier.

The weight of any evidence of malpractice — whether discovered through an out-of-court settlement or arbitration or a trial — should have

the same weight with the State Attorney General's Office as evidence from a trial to adjudicate punishment in medical malpractice cases. In my complaint to the Medical Board of California, Dr. Morton received a lower punishment since the evidence against him was not the result of a trial. That is not full justice for an injured patient and places a lesser emphasis on non-trial findings.

I favor a mechanism that would allow earlier findings by the Medical Board of California, so that they could be introduced in an active med mal legal case. In other words, earlier reporting say within 45 days after the medical malpractice was discovered or known by the perpetrators. The initial notification would be to the Department of Public Health and secondarily to the Medical Board of California where a preliminary investigation should be started.

A plaintiff's attorney is not concerned about how the Medical Board of California will rule against a defendant like Morton. That is strictly up to the injured patient. Armed with the knowledge that the Medical Board of California found gross negligence medical malpractice in my case and that the negligence caused me to be injured, I would have pressed my attorney to seek a much larger out-of-court settlement against Dr. Morton or a trial against him. Such a finding would be a heavy burden for a defendant to overcome.

As it stands, until the medical malpractice case is resolved, the Medical Board of California is not likely to conclude its investigation.

As far as periodic payments are concerned, the threshold should be raised from any amount over $50,000 to any amount over $250,000. If the settlement exceeds $250,000 a lump sum payment of $250,000 is paid at the time of the settlement. Injured plaintiffs need their money. It is ghoulish to string out payments to a plaintiff who may die and then let the payer off the hook by absolving him of liability when the patient dies. In practice, many cases settled for more than $50,000 are paid in full at the time of the settlement.

For future medical payments, the plaintiff should be allowed to choose a lump sum at time of settlement or be paid as expenses are incurred so that they will not be affected due to the affects of inflation over time on rising medical costs. A third alternative would be the purchase of a medical insurance policy for the injured plaintiff and an annuity to fund increased non-medical costs by the defendant(s).

I'd like to see an elective insurance policy made available to a patient or guardian of a patient prior to a serious medical procedure that would fund up to $20,000 to investigate a medical malpractice claim in case the outcome of the procedure is reported as medical malpractice. This way, more injured patients would have an avenue to seek justice for a medical malpractice injury if there is one.

I don't favor any changes to the fees attorneys get according to the statute.

The general populace of California needs a public information source about The MICRA and medical malpractice cases written at a twelfth to fourteenth grade level. That way, more people can understand what happens when you have a medical malpractice case. To people, information is power. In medical malpractice cases, the lawyers have the information — making the plaintiff less powerful, due to a lack of knowledge. This is wrong. The State of California needs to provide this.

I am not sure that raising the mandatory reporting threshold to the Medical Board of California from settlements exceeding $30,000 should be done. Medical practitioners who negligently injure patients within the State need to be under a bright spotlight.

Raising the mandatory minimum reporting threshold will likely increase the amounts doctors will agree to pay while not coming under scrutiny. This would be desirable, economically, for injured patients. Yet it could be bad for future patients who want to be aware of negligent physicians.

Leaving the standards as is won't necessarily aid patients who get injured in the future.

If all medical injury cases must be reported, then this becomes a moot point and the reporting threshold of any settlement over $30,000 disappears which would be a good idea.

I want the provision that allows defendant doctors to refuse to settle medical malpractice cases eliminated if they are covered by med mal insurance. The present statute gives them too much control and forces a plaintiff to go to trial.

I'd like to see a law that requires every healthcare institution or the office of any healthcare provider who provides patient care to post a notice for patients indicating where malpractice complaints can be filed with the State.

The MICRA has some significant shortcomings. What I've suggested might help remedy some of them.

So many people advocate keeping healthcare costs down by hammering medical malpractice settlements. What about the rising costs to the healthcare systems of new (and expensive) drugs and treatments? Folks, it's not all medical malpractice stuff. Yet, a medical malpractice cap for non-economic damages becomes the red-haired stepchild in the drama.

Raising the caps will ultimately raise the cost of medical care, as will enacting a "no-fault" system for claims below a certain dollar value. This is a given. How much healthcare costs increase? I do not know. I am the research staff for this book and I simply don't have the time or expertise to tell you that information.

In my mind, having been through a very painful malpractice, the increased cost is worth it in case a medical professional makes a significant preventable error in caring for you. And, it brings potential justice to more claims.

For other states who have already followed MICRA's lead, and for those who will follow California's lead with MICRA-type statutes, take note that MICRA is flawed and the ways that it is flawed. Under The MICRA, the words "and with liberty and justice for all" are not applicable.

Some people in the medical profession, the medical malpractice insurance profession and attorneys who defend those who have been sued under The MICRA or similar laws may not think too highly of me for what I have made public and for the changes I have suggested.

I say to them, too bad. The medical malpractice system in California — from the basic reporting all the way through the legal process — is lousy and needs meaningful reform for the masses. The time for meaningful reform is *now*.

This book puts the Governor of California and the California Legislature on notice to enact meaningful legislation to reform The MICRA and to create a system to adjudicate lower value medical malpractice claims.

That goes for other states who have patterned their med mal laws based on MICRA. In fact, it goes for every state legislator and every governor in each of our fifty states. The med mal laws in this country are sorely in need of reform.

For any federally elected official contemplating medical malpractice reform, I hope you have read this far in my book. If not, you need to read this book before you do something shallow regarding med mal reform. You need to grasp what is really going on with medical malpractice.

A Governor's task force of practicing attorneys and insurance economists can hammer out the necessary changes to MICRA and create a "no fault" system for lower value claims. Keep the politicians out of it.

If I could do it myself, I would.

In case the State Legislature does not want to effect changes to MICRA, a ballot initiative may be the only way. **Don't be surprised if you see one or more ballot initiatives about changing The MICRA in the 2014 State elections.**

This is where some eager law school students could make their bones. Start a grass roots movement and let the people vote on it.

Epilogue—The Aftermath

About the need to write this book...

In 2007, I decided to start reading everything in my legal file as a therapeutic exercise about my case. Then, after writing about the case, I decided to turn it into a book. My thought was that the tale might be worth telling so that some other people would not go into a medical malpractice case in California flying blind.

Mind you, for me, this was an arduous undertaking, given my history of PTSD. Plus, the subject matter was so distasteful. I abhorred penning the story as I had to re-live a situation that took a big chunk out of my life. Still, I pressed ahead.

Over time, I read everything including all the medical reports, the depositions, the medical records, the letters between Lobl and I, the medical bills — **everything.**

I received quite an education from what I read. By doing so, I felt that I finally understood from start to finish what had happened to me medically and legally.

I made a valiant attempt to complete a manuscript for publication. I worked at it for long hours over the course of seven months. It consumed me.

At that point, I found myself burned out emotionally and depressed recalling the story. I had a major depressive episode that lasted more than three months.

When that hit, I packed everything about my case in some storage boxes and put them in my garage where they would be out of my sight.

As I awaited a June 2011 arthroscopic shoulder procedure, medical personnel on the short-stay ward at VHMC reminded me of my past history of MRSA. They kept at it wanting me to wear isolation clothes.

Awful memories of March and April of 2004 were brought into my consciousness.

Finally, I had heard enough. I had an emotional meltdown in my room just prior to the procedure. At that point, I lashed out at several of the staff with profanity and pounding my fists on my bed. I remember screaming at one woman on the staff saying, "I'll show you MRSA!" as I bared the surgical scar on my chest from my aortic valve replacment surgery.

I later called the Head Nurse on the unit and the Infectious Disease Control Person for the hospital and complained about how insensitive the staff had been about the subject of MRSA with me.

Really though, they were just doing their jobs. It was me who was overly sensitive, not them. After all, they did not know what I had been through.

About two months post-surgery from the procedure, in August 2011, I decided that my anger level about my horrible MRSA infection was too high and not normal. I felt that it was time to do something about it.

I consulted with my psychiatric resident at the Sepulveda V.A. Medical Center, and he suggested that I write about it to release the anger and stress I felt about it. So, I did.

The result of those efforts is this book about my journey through the California medical malpractice system.

Once again, in writing the book, which is intended to be a case study, I sought to:

1. Share an actual medical malpractice case from a first person point of view

2. Detail what might happen in a medical malpractice case legally

3. Point out flaws in the laws governing medical malpractice cases

4. Suggest changes to medical malpractice laws that are sorely needed

5. Find some peace of mind for myself

Hopefully, in your minds, I've accomplished those goals. If not, the shortcomings are all mine. As far as finding some peace of mind, I am more at ease with what happened but I will never forget it.

Since I began writing the tale once again, I have mellowed out a great deal. In re-living some of the darkest days of my life in recalling what happened, the unpleasant thoughts that I dredged up dissipated — but not quickly. My mood swings were very unsettling. On some days, I had a nasty edge about the whole thing — just waiting to jump down someone's throat over the smallest thing.

With time, I've became much more at ease about the whole distasteful situation that almost did me in.

I was as honest and open in writing the story as I could be. It only took six years to complete this, from the time I initially wrote down my thoughts. I wrote it the way that it happened, even if it meant some of my thoughts were dark and raw and maybe not socially appropriate.

My mood is much better about the whole thing. I feel that I did what I thought was best for me during my entire journey, in spite of how I behaved at times.

I took note of how angry I was near the end of my med mal journey and realized that all of that was out of character for me. I knew that I had been pushed to my limits physically and emotionally for years. I saw that the anger I displayed was my "pop-off" valve opening to relieve emotional pressure, as opposed to keeping it all inside and facing the consequences of that.

In August 2012, I underwent a CT scan (using a radioactive isotope) of my thoracic area to determine the size of my aorta and whether or not any of my arteries in that area were blocked. This was after an echocardiogram indicated my aorta may have enlarged to the point that a surgical intervention was required to replace it.

The CT scan showed that my aorta had enlarged since the 2004 surgery but that it had been stable in size since measured in a 2010 CT scan. Because of that determination, no surgical intervention was necessary.

This does not rule out surgical intervention for me in the future.

Even so, I refuse to live my life with a dark cloud hanging over my head. I continue my bike rides and five-plus days per week in the gym. To me, this is the best defense I have, should I require future surgical intervention.

Remember, all of this was due to some preventable mistakes.

Lastly, I hope that none of you ever have an experience like the one I tried to recount in this book.

My final thought?

Consider this:

Two little boys, aged eight, were to be in a school play. One of the lines that the first little boy was to say was "Ha, Fair Maiden, I've come to fill your soul with hope."

The second little boy had one line in the play which was "Hark, a pistol shot" after a gun was fired off-stage.

On the night of the performance, the audience was filled with the parents of the students performing the play and other interested parties.

The boys were both anxious.

The curtain went up and the students began to speak.

On cue, the first little boy said, "Ha, Fair Maiden, I've come to fill your hole with soap."

The audience laughed and the first little boy's mom was aghast. This made the second little boy even more anxious.

A little later, on cue, just after a shot rang out off-stage, the second little boy said, "Hark, a shistol pot, errr a pissing pot, uhhh a postal... shit, oh, bullshit, I didn't want to be in this goddamn play anyway!"

Just like the second little boy in the joke, I didn't want to be in the goddamn play anyway!

End Notes

i. Nyman, John, "Cost of Screening Intensive Care Patients for Methicillin-Resistant Staphylococcus Aureus in Hospitals," *American Journal of Infection Control*, Vol. 39, Issue 1, pp. 27-34.

ii Eber, Michael, et al, "Clinical and Economic Outcomes Attributable to Health-Associated Sepsis and Pneumonia," *Archives of Internal Medicine*, Vol. 170, No. 4, February 22, 2010, pp. 347-353.

iii Savage, David G., "Obama's Talk of Medical Malpractice Reform Surprises Both Sides," *Los Angeles Times*, January 28, 2011.

iv Foreman, Tom, "2011 State of the Union: A Progress Report," *CNN Politics: Healthcare,* January 24, 2012.

v Brill, Steven, "Bitter Pill: Why Medical Care Costs Are Killing Us," *Time*, March 14, 2013.

vi Penycate, John, *The Tunnels of Cu Chi* (New York: Berkley Books, 1986), pp. 141-142.

vii Post-Traumatic Stress Disorder definition. United States Department of Veterans Affairs Center for PTSD.

viii Wikipedia, "*Staphylococcus aureus*," http://en.wikipedia.org/wiki/Staphylococcus_aureus, last accessed on April 29, 2013.

ix Deposition of Robert L. Shuman, MD, July 28, 2005, Long Beach, CA.

x Fox, Maggie, "Staph Bug Causes New Pneumonia," *Reuters*, January 9, 2007.

xi Moisse, Katie, "Antibiotic Resistance Could Bring 'End of Modern Medicine,'" ABC News "Medical Unit" Blog, March 16, 2012, last accessed April 29, 2013.

xii Wikipedia, "Infective endocarditis," http://en.wikipedia.org/wiki/Bacterial_endocarditis, last accessed on April 29, 2013.

xiii Gorwitz, R.J., et al., *Journal of Infectious Diseases* 2008, 197: 1226-34.

xivReuters News Service. "With Infections on Rise, Hospital Tactics Vary," *The Wall Street Journal*. December 26, 2005, p. D 5. http://www.hospitalinfection.org/dev/news%20articles/WSJ%20-%20Infections%20on%20Rise%20(12-26-06).pdf

xv Etienne, J. et. Al, "Instability of characteristics amongst coagulese-negative staphylococci causing endocarditis," *Journal of Medical Microbiology* 1990, Vol 32, pp. 115-122.

xvi Winer, John D., *De-Mystifying Medical Malpractice Cases—A Consumer Guide to Medical Malpractice Litigation* (Winer and McKenna, San Francisco, CA, 2004)

xvii Brown, Edmund G., "Statement of Former California Governor Jerry Brown Concerning MICRA," June 13, 1993, Nader.org, http://nader.org/wp-content/uploads/2012/10/JerryBrown-MICRA.pdf, last accessed May 9, 2013.

xviii Leubitz, Brian, "MICRA: Unaccountability by Another Name," CaliforniaProgressReport.com, January 19, 2011, http://www.californiaprogressreport.com/site/micra-unaccountability-another-name (website), last accessed May 9, 2013.

xix Hurt, Jr., James W. Hurt, Stolz and Cromwell, LLC blog of April 17, 2013 http://hurtstolz.com/medical-malpractice-wrongful-death-claims-approach-100000-a-year/ Last accessed May 20, 2013

xx "Preventable Harm: California Fails to Follow through with Patient Safety Laws," SafePatientProject.org, March 2010, http://www.safepatientproject.org/CAPatientSafetyReportFinal_2.pdf, last accessed May 12, 2013.

xxi Nunez, Daniela, "California Activists Urge Lawmakers to Reform California Medical Board," Blog of Daniela Nunez, SafePatientProject.org, March 22, 2013, http://safepatientproject.org/posts/4408-california-activists-urge-lawmakers-to-reform-california-medical-board, last accessed May 10, 2013.

xxii Ibid.

xxiii Brown, Eryn, "Medical Errors in Hospitals Go Undetected, Study Suggests," *The Los Angeles Times,* April 7, 2001, http://articles.latimes.com/2011/apr/07/news/la-heb-hospital-errors-20110407, last accessed May 10, 2013.

xxiv Kaplan, Karen, "Many Doctors Hide the Truth about Medical Errors, Study Finds," *The Los Angeles Times*, February 8, 20012, http://articles.latimes.com/2012/feb/08/news/la-heb-doctors-not-honest-with-patients-20120208, last accessed May 10, 2013.

xxv Terhune, Chad, "41% of California Hospitals Graded C or Lower on Patient Safety," *The Los Angeles Times,* June 6, 2012, http://articles.latimes.com/2012/jun/06/business/la-fi-hospital-safety-20120606, last accessed May 10, 2013.

xxvi Glover, Scott and Girion, Lisa, "Legal Drugs, Deadly Outcomes," *The Los Angeles Times,* November 11, 2012, http://www.latimes.com/news/science/prescription/la-me-prescription-deaths-20121111-html,0,2363903.htmlstory?main=true, last accessed on May 10, 2013.

xxvii Terhune, Chad, "UCLA Medical Center Gets Failing Grade on Patient Safety," *The Los Angeles Times,* November 28, 2012, http://articles.latimes.com/2012/nov/28/business/la-fi-ucla-hospital-grade-20121128, last accessed May 10, 2013.

xxviii Join Together Staff "California Legislators: Use Database to Find Doctors who Overprescribe Painkillers." The Partnership at Drugfree.org March 13, 2013 www.drugfree.org/ Last accessed May 20, 2013

xxix Price, Jr., Curren D. and Gordon, Richard S., Letter to Sharon Levine, MD, April 1, 2013.

xxx 38IsTooLateLate on Facebook, July 1, 2013

xxxi "Advocates and Victims Thank Senate Leader for Holding Hearings on 38 Year Old Damage Cap Law to Address CA Patient Safety Crisis" http://www.consumerwatchdog.org/newsrelease/advocates-and-victims-thank-senate-leader-holding-hearings-38-year-old-damage-cap-law-ad

xxxii Davis, Richard (host), "AfterWords: Marty Makary," C-SPAN's *BookTV,* December

2012, http://www.booktv.org/Watch/14026/After+Words+Marty+Makary+Unaccountabl e+What+Hospitals+Wont+Tell+You+and+How+Transparency+Can+Revolutionize+H ealth+Care+hosted+by+Richard+Davis+Sibley+Memorial+Hospital+President.aspx, last accessed on May 11, 2013.

[xxxiii] Makary, Marty, "How to Stop Hospitals from Killing Us," *The Wall Street Journal*, September 21, 2012, http://online.wsj.com/article/SB10000872396390444620104578008263334441352 .html, last accessed May 10, 2013.

[xxxiv] Feinstein, Dianne, "Statement of Senator Dianne Feinstein 'On the OB/GYN Medical Malpractice Reform Bill,'" Congressional Record Vol. 150 No. 20, February 24, 2004, Washington, DC.

[xxxv] Diamond, Dan, "Why We Can't Get National Malpractice Reform," California Healthline, February 1, 2012, http://www.californiahealthline.org/road-to-reform/2012/why-we-cant-get-national-malpractice-reform.aspx, last accessed May 11, 2013.

[xxxvi] Pace, Nicholas, et al, "Capping Non-Economic Awards in Medical Malpractice Trials: California Jury Verdicts under MICRA," The Rand Corporation, Santa Monica, CA, Monograph, 2004.

[xxxvii] Pace, Nicholas, et al, "Changing the Medical Malpractice Debate: What have we learned from California's MICRA?" The Rand Corporation, Santa Monica, CA, Arlington, VA, and Pittsburgh, PA, January 12, 2012.

[xxxviii] Hamm, William G., et al, "California's MICRA Reforms: Increasing the Cap on Non-Economic Damages Would Increase the Cost of and Reduce Access to Healthcare," February 2005.

[xxxix] Hamm, William G. et al. *MICRA Lowers Healthcare Costs, Ensuring Patients Have Access to Healthcare*. LECG, November 2008.

[xl] Stone, Kimberly "CJAC Supports President's Support of Medical Malpractice Reform." CJAC January 26, 2011 January 26, 2011 CJAC.org Last accessed May 20, 2013

[xli] Join Staff "CJAC Files Amicus Brief Against Latest Appeal to Overturn MICRA." November 12, 2010 http://cjac.org Last accessed May 20, 2013

[xlii] Gallegos, Alicia "California's Non-economic Damages Cap Upheld." September 26, 2011 Amednews.com Last accessed May 20, 2013

[xliii] Yeung, Bernice "State's Medical Malpractice Law Faces More Challenges." July 2, 2012 CaliforniaWatch.org Las accessed May 20, 2012

[xliv] Lefler, Rebecca A. *Application for Leave to File Amici Curiae Brief in Support of Bernard Millman et al.* Tucker and Ellis, LLP March 6, 2013 ama-assn.org Last accessed May 20, 2013

[xlv] Yeung, Bernice "State's Medical Malpractice Law Faces More Challenges." July 2, 2012 CaliforniaWatch.org Las accessed May 20, 2012

[xlvi] Diamond, Dan, "Why We Can't Get National Malpractice Reform," California Healthline, February 1, 2012, http://www.californiahealthline.org/road-to-reform/2012/why-we-cant-get-national-malpractice-reform.aspx, last accessed

May 11, 2013.

xlvii Nader, Ralph, "Nader Calls on Governor Brown to Rescind Cap on Medical Injury Compensation," October 11, 2012, naderorg.com, http://nader.org/2012/10/10/nader-calls-on-gov-jerry-brown-to-recind-cap-on-medical-injury-compensation/, last accessed on May 12, 2013.

xlviii Baker, Tom, *The Medical Malpractice Myth* (University of Chicago Press: Chicago and London, 2005).

xlix Baker, Tom, *The Medical Malpractice Myth* (University of Chicago Press: Chicago and London, 2005), pp. 158-180.

l Landro, Laura, "Doctors Learn to Say 'I'm Sorry,'" *The Wall Street Journal,* January 24, 2007, p. D5, http://online.wsj.com/article/SB116960074741385710.html, last accessed May 13, 2013.

www.ingramcontent.com/pod-product-compliance
Lightning Source LLC
Chambersburg PA
CBHW051441170526
45166CB00001B/66

*9 781484 870297 *